Praise for **Co-Regulation Handbook**

"In this book, Ms. Murphy explains co-regulation as a way of being with, doing together, and teaching children with learning challenges. Instead of the adult directing and prompting the child through endless steps of an activity, a common method that can quickly become frustrating for all involved, with a co-regulation approach, the adult sets up activities such that the child has a specific role, one in which they are competent, and through this role the child, from the start, successfully participates in the whole, meaningful activity, and—and perhaps most importantly—participates in *harmony together* with the adult. More learning comes through creating alterations to the child's role (e.g., swapping roles), or adding complexity to the role or to the activity itself. In this way adults expand children's competence through meaningful participation and from a place of harmonious interaction. Activities included as examples are as disparate as cooking, playing games, and playdates. As in her *Declarative Language Handbook*, Ms. Murphy presents complex material with clarity and compelling, illustrative examples. This book will be invaluable for parents as well as teachers, and therapists across disciplines."

-Karen Levine, Ph.D., Psychologist
Lecturer on Psychiatry, Harvard Medical School

"Co-Regulation Handbook provides logical and functional strategies for helping us 'walk with' kids on the path of independence instead of pulling or pushing them! This Handbook provides simple and logical strategies for effectively teaching students to value themselves and others within the social world. Simply brilliant!"

-Beckham Linton MA, CCC-SLP
Social Cognitive Coach, www.heartlandsociallearning.com

"When *Declarative Language Handbook* came out I recommended the book to my Facebook and YouTube followers, many of whom shared with me how grateful they were for recommending the book to them. I will be doing the same with *Co-Regulation Handbook*. The brilliance of Linda's writing is her ability to make concepts practical and she provides clear and concise directions regarding how to implement strategies. Linda's voice fills a tremendous need in the ADHD world, which for decades has ignored the incredibly important role language plays in building skills. Like *Declarative Language Handbook*, I consider this book a necessity for parents of kids with ADHD."

-Ryan Wexelblatt, LCSW, ADHD-CCSP (ADHD Dude)

"Relationship is the key to unlocking true reciprocal communication, intrinsic motivation, and a strong sense of self. Linda Murphy's companion books, *Declarative Language Handbook* and *Co-regulation Handbook*, are clear, concise and communicate core principles of person-centered care I find foundational in my work. I will be reaching for and promoting these two books often to support the families I serve."

-Sherri Miller, MS, CCC-SLP,
Founder of Communicating Potential LLC

"Linda does an amazing job of explaining what co-regulation is and how to implement it when working with children. This book is so user friendly—providing examples, games, and stories that are so relatable. Linda does a great job connecting the dots to help readers understand how co-regulation relates to many other important aspects of life such as self-regulation, executive functioning and creating meaningful social experiences. Using co-regulation during my occupational therapy sessions has helped me make better connections and relationships with the children that I treat. Each relationship has been formed in such a fluid and natural way - it feels so balanced. Such a great read, I can't wait to recommend this book to the families that I work with in the future!"

-Brooke Belmonte, Occupational Therapist MS, OTR/LC

"This book is a beautifully written guide on how to form a deep, meaningful and impactful partnership with your child. This is important for any child, but when your child experiences the world differently this partnership is invaluable. I have watched my son (and myself!) grow in so many ways since we started practicing co-regulation with Linda, and I feel so much more equipped to help him navigate a world that can be confusing and scary to him. As we navigate together, he is learning skills he will use his whole life, and I am learning how to be a better teacher! This book will help guide parents and caregivers, and will explain step by step how to turn everyday moments into learning opportunities. These moments will turn into a way of being that will leave child and caregiver feeling empowered and competent, and for us that has been incredibly rewarding.

In this book Linda will walk you through the process of learning about co-regulation in an easy to read and fun way. Working with Linda has been life changing for us, and I am so happy she wrote this book so I can share with others what has been working so well for us. Every adult who works with a child who has social learning differences has an opportunity to make this incredible connection we have found through co-regulation.

This book is a MUST READ, the knowledge in these pages will help transform the child's experience and set the stage to learn and grow together in a positive and meaningful way."

-Charlie's Mom

"A few months ago I said, in reference to Linda Murphy's Declarative Language Handbook, that it would be "the most important book on the shelves of clinicians and parents." While I stand by this statement I am adapting and signaling that there are now two most-important handbooks.

Parents and professionals alike will be pleased by the conceptual dove-tailing of Declarative Language and Co-Regulation. The writing is scientifically elegant and the theoretical underpinnings come alive through illustrative examples and easily applied real-life activities."

-Rachelle K. Sheely, Ph.D.
President RDIconnect, Inc

Co-Regulation Handbook

Creating Competent, Authentic Roles
for Kids with Social Learning Differences,
So We All Stay Positively Connected
Through the Ups and Downs of Learning

Linda K. Murphy MS, CCC-SLP

First paperback edition February 2021

Book design by Brent Spears

ISBN 978-1-7345162-2-7 (paperback)
ISBN 978-1-7345162-3-4 (ebook)

Library of Congress Control Number: 2021902798

www.co-regulation.com

DEDICATION

This one is for my Dad, Paul E. Murphy. Thank you for all that you do for me, every day. ♥

Contents

ACKNOWLEDGEMENTS

I'd like to express gratitude to Dr. Steven Gutstein, Dr. Rachelle Sheely, and to the Relationship Development Intervention® (RDI) community that they have created over the past 20+ years. Dr. Gutstein's and Dr. Sheely's guidance and wisdom concerning how kids learn—especially kids with social learning differences—helped me discover whom I wanted to be as a therapist, teacher, and parent. Within the RDI Community I have learned—and continue to learn—about co-regulation and declarative language, among many other things. Understanding these concepts grounds my teaching every day.

I'd also like to thank my family—Rob, and my busy, lovable boys, Freddie and Desmond! They continually support me in my work as a writer and clinician, while also giving me many (many!) opportunities to put into practice what I preach. Practicing co-regulation and declarative language daily is a lot harder as a parent than a clinician… Thank you for teaching me that!

I am so appreciative to the families who have allowed me to share our work together and their stories in this book. I cherish our relationships and I learn so much from all of you.

I am forever grateful to my team at Peer Projects Therapy From the Heart because they too are the ones that put these important ideas into practice every day. You are all stars! And, to my good friend and cheerleader, Amanda Hynes… thank you for continually (gently) pushing me outside of my comfort zone and helping me find creative ways to keep sharing my work.

INTRODUCTION

Why Are We Here (Again)?

In my first book, Declarative Language Handbook, I shared my first passion—declarative language. This is a thoughtful speaking style that helps kids with social learning differences feel competent, connected, and understood. I knew I wanted to write more, and some readers even asked me to provide activities to target the areas of social learning that I discussed in my first book. I thought about this idea but couldn't quite move forward.

Declarative language has an important partner called co-regulation that is equally important to use and understand when helping kids with social learning differences feel competent, connected, and understood.

As I thought about why I was stalled, I realized it was because there was still more to teach on the ground level. I use declarative language constantly, but it is not the only tool in my toolbox. In fact, declarative language has an important partner called co-regulation that is equally important to use and understand when helping

3

kids with social learning differences feel competent, connected, and understood.

As with declarative language, I learned first about co-regulation when training to become a Relationship Development Intervention® (RDI) consultant. And, as with declarative language, once I understood it—what it looked like, what it felt like, and its purpose—it changed everything I did. Declarative language is a way of speaking, and co-regulation is a way of *being*.

Declarative language is a way of speaking, and co-regulation is a way of *being*.

Co-regulation establishes a shared focus of attention with our communication partner. In other words, we both know we are thinking about the same thing at the same time. As a result, it helps us feel certain of our connection in the moment. When two people with different social learning styles are together, there is often a disconnect between what each person is attending to. We might be together physically, but we are thinking about different things. Additionally, sometimes we are not together in thought because the other person's pace is faster than ours, or because our pace is faster than theirs.

Understanding and practicing co-regulation helps us stay together in our thoughts and actions. It works toward maintaining a unified pace so that no one is left behind. It grounds us in what we are doing together right now and lays the foundation for all that follows—authentic social connections, reciprocity, conversation that is mutually meaningful, and ultimately, an understanding of our community and world.

Co-regulation starts early in development, but when a child and caregiver have different learning styles, vary in their attentional patterns (i.e. their attentional capacity and what they attend to), or when one experiences anxiety about new things, the result is that this duo of communication partners do not get the same practice and opportunities with co-regulation as others who are more naturally in sync.

But just like with declarative language, it is never too late to start. What co-regulation looks like between a young child and caregiver may be different than what it looks like between an older child and caregiver, but you can always go back and develop this skill together.

Co-regulation, along with declarative language, is my foundation when helping to develop social competence and success between communication partners. I rarely use one without the other. My goal in this book is to teach you the concept of co-regulation because it has been so important to me. I want to teach you what it is, how it feels, how to know when you have it, and to recognize when you don't. Breakdowns in co-regulation are natural and expected, not something to avoid or fear. And as you notice breakdowns in co-regulation with your child, I want you to also become competent and confident in navigating repairs.

The idea of co-regulation has been around for a long time, and I continue to hear more people talking about it. Because it took me years to deeply appreciate what this term means, I know others might welcome an easy to understand explanation and ideas for application all in one place.

My goal in this book is to help anyone who cares about someone with social learning differences—parents, grandparents, teachers, therapists, babysitters, etc.—understand co-regulation so they can use it to strengthen their social connection with that individual and create a positive learning environment.

My goal in this book is to help anyone who cares about someone with social learning differences—parents, grandparents, teachers, therapists, babysitters, etc.—understand co-regulation so they can use it to strengthen their social connection with that individual and create a positive learning environment.

Finally, as with my last book, I will do my best to honor the time you are giving me and keep this book practical, user friendly, and to the point. Let's go!

A note about how to use this book...

As with *Declarative Language Handbook*, this book is meant to be practical. You can read the chapters in order or just read chapters that are the most meaningful to you.

Having said that, everyone should read Chapter 2, because this will let you know what you can do right away to start putting co-regulation into practice in your everyday life.

If you are interested in diving deeper into the relationships between co-regulation and the areas of self-regulation, conversation, and executive function, continue right into the three chapters in Part 2 after you finish Chapter 2.

In Part 3, I provide more technical information around the mechanics of co-regulation, how you may apply what you are learning across different contexts or situations, and how to adjust complexity as you go. Adjusting complexity means simplifying what you are doing when something is too hard for your child or adding challenge when something is too easy! You will want to know how to adjust what you are doing to keep everyone competent and successful, so these chapters are important to get to as you are ready.

Chapter 1: Why Are We Here (Again)?

Part 4 is also essential for your learning, so be sure not to skip this information on pacing and troubleshooting. Breakdowns in co-regulation are to be expected, and self-monitoring our own pace is essential. These chapters will give you important food for thought and strategies for when you feel stuck.

I imagine many readers will be interested in learning how to apply co-regulation to peer interactions. I have dedicated Part 5 to this topic, which includes a framework for establishing positive peer interactions as well as how to think about competitive games.

In Part 6, I provide practice sets to help you become comfortable applying ideas of co-regulation across range of opportunities.

In Part 7, I review how to notice progress over time and I share a snapshot of some existing research.

In Chapter 15, I end with my vision for the future and what I hope to change with how we teach our kids who have social learning differences.

CHAPTER 2:

What You Need to Know to Get Started Right Away

For those of you eager to get started, I offer this chapter to share the basics in terms of what co-regulation is and how to establish it with your child. As with declarative language, all that I have learned about co-regulation comes from the RDI community. Although I have heard more people speaking about co-regulation recently, my education on this topic began within RDI. I continue to learn about it, explore ideas and understand it on deeper levels from my fellow RDI Consultants.

Interactions are not predetermined but are the fluid, ongoing and unfolding process of continuous reciprocal communicative exchanges between individuals.

In a nutshell, establishing co-regulation means that two people—for example, a child and a caregiver—are partners in an interaction in which they are responding contingently to each other moment-to-moment. Interactions are not predetermined (for example as a script in a theater production might be) but are the fluid, ongoing, and unfolding process of continuous reciprocal communicative exchanges between individuals. In addition, there is balance; each person contributes equally to the exchange. Co-regulation is not a recipe but a dance, and when two individuals have different social learning styles, it can be hard to achieve this for several reasons. But it is worth it to learn how to because so much positive, interpersonal learning happens when true co-regulation is the backdrop.

Now, I will take a step back and explain how to construct co-regulatory opportunities so it feels less elusive and more attainable.

Having roles of this nature (competent, authentic, contingent) lays the groundwork for mutual appreciation, respect, and care.

First, to achieve a balance, both individuals must have competent, authentic, and contingent roles within the interaction. Having roles of this nature (competent, authentic, contingent) lays the groundwork for mutual appreciation, respect, and care. Each of these three elements is critical for co-regulation, so I will go through each one individually as it relates to a child and caregiver, and daily routines.

1. **Competent role** – This simply means, is the role you are assigning the child a competent one for them at that moment in time? If they are competent in that role, this means they can do it on their own, without prompting, when given time. Example: a competent role for a 9-month-old might be to bring a bottle to their mouth because at that point in development, they usually no longer need their caregiver to hold the bottle in place. A competent role for many 11-year-old children might be to push a shopping cart down the aisle of a grocery store. In contrast, this latter example would probably not be a competent role for a 3 or 4-year-old.

2. **Authentic role** – This means the role is real and meaningful versus contrived. Kids can spot the difference! As we will get

9

into, some of the best opportunities for co-regulation are daily activities around the house that parents typically do on their own. These tasks need to get done no matter what, so when a child joins in, they feel and observe how their contributions are making a difference for their family. Examples might be helping with recycling or laundry, or helping to bake.

3. **Contingent role** – This means the process is done in partnership. The child has a role, the caregiver has a role, and both roles are needed to get the job done. If one person does not do their part, the activity or process will not move forward. This is where we start to get at a meaningful connection between two individuals. Examples of contingent roles using the ideas above might be:

   - *Baby bottle*
     Role 1: Caregiver prepares the bottle and places it on the highchair tray and then…
     Role 2: The baby brings it up to their mouth.

   - *Grocery shopping*
     Role 1: Caregiver chooses items on the shelves at the grocery store and places them in the cart while…
     Role 2: The child pushes the cart alongside them.

   - *Recycling*
     Role 1: A child takes one side of the recycling bin while…
     Role 2: Their caregiver takes the other side, and together they walk it to the curb.

   - *Laundry*
     Role 1: Caregiver takes an item out of the dryer and hands it to their child, and…
     Role 2: The child then places it in the laundry basket.

- *Baking*
  Role 1: Caregiver pours the allotted amount of flour or sugar into a measuring cup, and...
  Role 2: The child then dumps it into the bowl.

There are so many ways to create competent, authentic, and contingent roles in our daily routines, and therefore engage kids in co-regulatory opportunities. An important first step is to view daily routines or tasks as opportunities for social engagement and to then look at these through the lens of competent roles. As you start to think about opportunities for your child, think through how you might carve out a competent role for them. Approach the activity thinking about what the best and most successful role for your child would be. Remember, in that role they will be independent, as long as you give them the time that they need.

An important first step is to view daily routines or tasks as opportunities for social engagement and to then look at these through the lens of competent roles.

It is also helpful to think of co-regulation in terms of actions. Of course, we all want kids to become competent and skilled conversationalists when interacting with a range of communication partners. But what is important to appreciate is that establishing reciprocity, or the give and take needed for meaningful conversation, does not need to start with words. In fact, developmentally, reciprocity starts with actions. Therefore, with co-regulation, it makes sense to start with actions as well.

As we help kids engage in an activity, where they have competent, authentic, contingent roles in an ongoing way, or where co-regulation is sustained over increased periods of time, they learn how to stay

11

engaged in the reciprocal flow of social interactions. You will come to see how although this may start with seemingly simple roles (carrying out a recycling bin together), over time these can be expanded to include more complex roles and more reciprocal opportunities.

If you read my first book, *Declarative Language Handbook*, you may remember Eliza and Christopher. I want to share stories with you about their introduction to co-regulation, in order to provide more examples, illustrating how it all works.

I first taught Eliza's parents about co-regulation when she was three years old. Before understanding this framework, her parents' play activities were more open ended, and they playfully entertained her to sustain engagement. For example, I have one clip that I share often where Eliza's father is tickling her and picking her up over his shoulders, and another where Eliza's mother is drumming alongside her, playfully trying to secure her attention. In each, Eliza shifts her attention to her parents for brief moments. For example, she laughs with her dad, and she visually references what her mother is doing. In each of these scenarios though, Eliza is more of a passive observer in the routines—watching or being entertained. She is not authentically involved or provided a competent role.

However, once her parents learned about co-regulation, we thought of daily tasks in which they could comfortably include her as a partner and assign her a competent role. Her dad thought to include her as his partner in getting some boxes ready for recycling. He lined them up on the kitchen floor, with the intention of stacking them inside each other by size. He pointed to each box as he needed it, thoughtfully guiding her attention, and Eliza would hand it to him. At that point in time, being the "box hander" was a competent role for Eliza, while her father was the "box stacker." And what was observed in those moments was authentic, enjoyable teamwork between a father and daughter.

With Eliza's mother, she chose sweeping up pine needles off the floor around Christmas time for co-regulation practice. She handed Eliza the dustpan to hold ("dustpan holder") while she swept ("sweeper"). Once Eliza had enough pine needles in the dustpan, her mother guided her to dump them in a small cardboard box. As they worked together and Eliza sustained attention and engagement to their shared activity, her mother decided she could swap roles with Eliza, and Eliza would remain competent. So, they swapped; Eliza became the "sweeper", and her mother became the "dustpan holder." Her mother recognized that because this was a new task for Eliza, she needed to start by offering her the simpler role of "dustpan holder." If she had invited her to sweep first, before Eliza had really had a chance to observe and learn the process, it probably would not have been a competent role for her. Her mother set her up for success, and then added challenge by swapping roles as Eliza was ready.

With both processes, Eliza's parents slowed their pace, ensuring that she completed her designated part before they moved ahead. They moved along in the process, moment-to-moment, adjusting and attending to each other, and working to stay in sync as they accomplished their shared goals. This was quite different from the previous clips where Eliza's attention to her parents was fragile.

Eliza and her parents moved along in the process, moment-to-moment, adjusting and attending to each other, and working to stay in sync as they accomplished their shared goals.

I also want to provide some examples for a young adult. I talked a bit about Christopher and Judy in my first book and I will continue to share stories about them in this book. Christopher is a young autistic man, and Judy, his mother had come to me to find ways to deepen their communication and find greater opportunities for them to connect. As Judy learned about the idea of co-regulation, she came up with some solid authentic and meaningful roles for Christopher within activities that they could do together.

I remember in one video Judy showed me, they raked leaves together. Judy raked leaves into a pile, and Christopher's role was to pick up the leaves and place them in a trash barrel. They continued this over several minutes, as Christopher observed Judy bring the leaves to him in a pile and he placed them where they went, happy and proud to join her in this work. Another example was when Judy needed to carry a chair upstairs. She saw this as an opportunity for co-regulation and invited Christopher and his cousin to carry the chair together; Christopher took one side of the chair and his cousin took the other.

As you may notice from this example, co-regulation is always a great framework within which to create balanced peer interaction opportunities as well. It is a positive, natural way for two people to connect around a joint focus of attention, work towards a common goal, and form a shared memory together.

You may also notice co-regulation is all about the moments. We are not necessarily looking for an activity that extends over a long period of time, especially when starting out. Rather, we are on the lookout for the small moments that happen in our day, that we can optimize for social connection and learning when we view them in a slightly different way.

We are on the lookout for the small moments that happen in our day, that we can optimize for social connection and learning when we view them in a slightly different way.

Here are two more things to keep in mind as you begin to think about co-regulation and creating these types of opportunities with kids:

1. **Enter with a guiding, invitational mindset, using declarative language.** It is critical that the child is not directed or prompted to "do co-regulation" but rather that they are invited to join in a shared process. Parents are often skeptical at first that their child will join on their own. However, what is great to see is how kids usually do join when they know they can be competent, and how they stay connected as long as those feelings of competence and contribution sustain.

2. **With any of these co-regulatory opportunities, the task or activity that you are doing is secondary and merely a backdrop for creating a positive engagement and connection over time.** Keep in mind the words "process over product." It is most important that the child is a true partner and competent. This often requires us to slow our pace, so the child has the time they need to notice, initiate, and respond in an ongoing way. If you are in a rush or feel it will be too hard for you to slow down within a specific activity, then it is not a good time to practice co-regulation. As with declarative language, choose a time that you can focus on the process of what you are doing together and not worry about finishing a product. For example, it may not be a good time to first practice co-regulation when you are trying to get out the door in the morning. Or it is okay if you can only practice co-regulation for part of your laundry routine rather than all of it. Keep in mind Eliza and her mom as an example: the process of "sweeping together" and staying in sync was more important than the product of the floor being clean.

Hopefully, that is enough to help you start thinking in a new way! I'll have more nuts, bolts, and frameworks to help you think about and create opportunities for co-regulation in Part 3: Mechanics.

PART 2:

CO-REGULATION: THE FOUNDATION OF SOCIAL CONNECTION

CHAPTER 3:
Managing Ourselves: How are Self-Regulation and Co-Regulation Related?

You may have heard the terms self-regulation and co-regulation, but not have been able to figure out what they mean and what the difference is. I want to explain these to you in my own words, through the lens of social communication. I know an occupational therapist would be able to provide more technical details and nuances related to self-regulation, and there are many resources listed in the bibliography for those that want to dive deep into that topic specifically. But, for my purposes, I want to help you understand these terms in relation to social development, and how I use and think about these concepts when I'm supporting kids to be stronger and more independent communicators. Here goes...

Self-regulation is the process of managing yourself! And there is a lot we need to manage every day. We need to manage our physical needs (hunger, thirst, fatigue, need to move, need to go to the bathroom, etc.) and we need to manage our emotions—both big and small. When we self-regulate successfully, we are in control of our body. We can make good decisions in the moment, recognize our internal needs, and respond to our emotions in adaptive ways. For example, we may feel worried or frustrated or scared or mad or excited, but we are still in control of our actions and words, whatever they might be. When someone struggles with self-regulation, they may appear impulsive, have a meltdown when upset, or perhaps become paralyzed with worry in certain situations. As we get older and our nervous systems mature, we all get better at self-regulating because we learn what will help us personally to manage our needs.

Now, let's think about the development of self-regulation. Developmentally, babies and young children need help regulating. Youngsters do not yet have the skills to manage their physical states or their big emotions on their own. This is expected. They need their caregivers to help read their cues and emotions, and to provide what is needed. This may be food, a diaper change, a hug, or even some kind words. For babies, their needs might be obvious. The baby cries and the caregiver often intuitively knows whether to feed them, put them down for a nap, or change their diaper. As kids grow, caregivers are still needed. For example, think about how a parent may help their child manage big feelings of excitement when waiting for their birthday party to start, or manage their scared feelings if they see a bee, or manage their feelings of pain after falling off their bike. Caregivers even help kids manage their hurt feelings when another child has been unkind. There is a lot going on there!

Kids need caregivers to help them regulate. When a caregiver responds contingently, in the moment, to a child's need or cues, this is an example of co-regulation: *I am helping you regulate. We are regulating together. We are regulating as a team because I know you can't yet do it all on your own. You are upset, and I respond contingently by comforting you in a way I know will help you personally.*

Kids need caregivers to help them regulate. When a caregiver responds contingently, in the moment, to a child's need or cues, this an example of co-regulation.

Now let's think about kids with social learning differences. Self-regulation can be challenging! We know this to be true. These kids might struggle to read their own internal cues and have trouble managing big emotions such as worry, frustration, and excitement. We may see reactions that look big from our perspective or observe impulsive actions as a result. Because they are struggling to manage their big emotions and internal needs, they cannot always respond in adaptive, thoughtful ways.

Yet this is what we want kids to do. And, as they get older, caregivers, teachers, family members, etc. may become impatient when kids are not able to regulate. Especially when we think they should be able to because of their age. We then might place behavioral expectations on them or deliver consequences for not getting it together, even though developmentally they may not be able to do it. These strategies may help at times, but when a child continues to struggle with regulating, co-regulation is a better and more positive approach to use.

By slowing down to engage kids in a competent role that is contingent on yours, you will help ground them in the moment, learn more about the situation from their perspective, figure out what may feel hard or scary or upsetting to them, and from that place of mutual understanding, guide their overall learning.

Co-regulation is a natural, guiding, and supportive way to help kids regulate when they cannot yet do so independently. By slowing down to engage them in a competent role that is contingent on yours, you will help ground them in the moment, learn more about the situation from their perspective, figure out what may feel hard or scary or upsetting to them, and from that place of mutual understanding, guide their overall learning.

For example, imagine a child being invited to join an activity with others. Interpersonal communication by its nature is dynamic. Although there is some predictability, we don't always know exactly what the other person is going to say or do. Uncertainty can cause feelings of worry or anxiety for kids with social learning differences. Worry and anxiety are feelings that can get pretty big and be difficult for a child to manage on their own. Therefore, we may see kids shut down or say no to social interactions or activities that feel scary to them.

If we understand this, that the child is feeling worried in response to the uncertainty, and that they are having trouble managing this worry on their own, we can approach them with understanding and create opportunities for co-regulation and competence. This will help them engage and regulate, and ultimately help them feel comfortable doing that new thing both in the present and in future opportunities.

Co-regulation is a positive way to help kids regulate while becoming proficient in something new. It is a positive backdrop that invites kids to engage in a way that helps them feel safe, connected, competent, and challenged at a manageable pace.

Co-regulation is a positive way to help kids regulate while becoming proficient in something new. Co-regulation is a positive, supportive backdrop that invites kids to engage in a way that helps them feel safe, connected, competent, and challenged at a manageable pace. It is a strategy that feels so much better than punitive consequences for what appears to be bad behavior (or punishing a child's inability to self-regulate). Co-regulation helps the activity or interaction start in a positive, fluid way, and helps the child stay connected as things get underway, and as a result - everyone feels better.

Here are a few specific examples of how to do this when emotions are escalating.

Imagine inviting your child to play a new game. They say no. Instead of pushing harder or giving up completely, you then offer a co-regulatory partnership: *I have an idea! We'll be a team. You can be the spinner and I'll be the game piece mover.* They may be more likely to join because this setup feels less scary.

Or when your child is resisting starting homework. *How about to get started, you be the idea guy, and I'll be the writer. You say what you're thinking, and I'll help us get it down on paper.* You help the child initiate the task by sharing the work, because you realize that doing all of it at once was not a competent role for them at that moment in time. Once the process is underway, you can fade back and allow the child greater independence.

Or for an art project that a child may feel unsure of given the fine motor demands involved, you might try, *How about this? You can be the marker chooser, and I'll be the color-er to start.* Then, as the child feels comfortable, you could swap roles or invite them to color a portion of the picture, and expand their role as you sense they are ready.

All these opportunities create positive partnerships instead of power struggles and increase the likelihood that the child will feel comfortable enough to join.

Here is a real example that illustrates how kids may try to use co-regulation to calm worries. I observed this event when visiting one of my clients in his classroom several years ago. At the time, it became clear that the school and I were wearing vastly different

21

lenses when it came to regulation, and I had wished the child's teachers knew about co-regulation.

Teddy, who was eight at the time, was feeling anxious—probably about many things, but one specific thing that I recall was that his teachers were getting ready for a drill of some sort. There had been an announcement over the loudspeaker telling teachers to get ready. As a visitor to the school, I didn't completely understand what was happening, but I observed them lower the blinds, close the door, and turn off the lights, without explanation to Teddy.

As they made these quiet changes in the environment, the teachers worked to keep students on task with their academics. Teddy is a child who asks questions, and often asks the same questions over and over. In my time with him, I have come to understand that his question asking is often a sign of anxiety. When he is feeling especially anxious, his number of questions increase.

Unfortunately, his teachers viewed this pattern of question asking in a behavioral way. They talked about Teddy getting stuck on irrelevant topics. It made me incredibly sad at the time that they could not see how Teddy was feeling and that his question asking was his attempt to co-regulate. He was searching for a trusted adult to help him feel better by engaging in a predictable question/answer routine, or by engaging in a reciprocal exchange where he had a competent role.

I also viewed him as desperately seeking social connection in that moment. Often his questions were about his teacher's personal life. For example, he was curious to learn more about her friends or home life. In the moment, I observed his teachers ignore his questions, because they were viewed as "off task," and attempt to redirect his attention to schoolwork. And they did so without acknowledging his communication in the moment. As an observer to the classroom,

I was not allowed to speak to anyone so I couldn't share what I was thinking until later. But this sequence of events broke my heart.

Now, let me be clear. I understand that at times we need to help kids attend to their work and help them hold their thoughts to stay on track and get things done. But this was different. This was a child feeling incredibly anxious who was desperately trying to regulate, but he needed help from his teachers to do so. He could not, in that moment, self-regulate independently because his feelings of worry were too big. And his teachers were not reading or responding to these cues.

I saw a child trying to connect and trying to co-regulate to help manage his feelings of worry amidst unexplained changes in the environment. His teachers saw him using a behavior that they wanted to extinguish. I am including this example because we must do better. It is not just on kids to regulate and do all the work. Sometimes they truly need our help, and we do them a disservice when we ignore their attempts to get it.

It is not just on kids to regulate and do all the work. Sometimes they truly need our help, and we do them a disservice when we ignore their attempts to get it.

I want educators out there to think differently when kids ask questions repeatedly. View this as communication that they are using, perhaps to connect, but also perhaps to help themselves regulate. Take it as an opportunity to provide comfort and reassurance when that is called for, and to build trust. Instead of ignoring or redirecting without explanation, use co-regulation to help ease the child's worries or fears, and then together over time, work to help them find strategies that they can use independently to calm. In this example, the teachers could have also followed up his questions with declarative language providing information about what was going on. For example, *Teddy, I'm so happy you want to learn more about me! But I'm also wondering if you are feeling worried about something... Let's figure out what we can to do help you feel better, so you feel comfortable getting back to your schoolwork.*

In summary, using co-regulation is a positive way to invite and engage a child in an activity that they may not yet feel competent in. It is also a way to help kids ease their worries or fear, especially when these feelings are too big for them to manage on their own. As kids regulate to you, you will be helping them manage their feelings of uncertainty, and subsequently increasing their ability to self-regulate.

Kids needs to be able to self-regulate to be successful social communicators as they grow, and co-regulation helps them get there.

CHAPTER 4:

Creating and Sustaining Authentic Reciprocity: From Co-Regulation to Conversation

As discussed in the previous chapter, co-regulation supports over-all regulation. When a child is regulated, they are better able to attend to a shared focus of interest and be thoughtful in how they respond to information in their environment. What I'd like to talk about in this chapter is how co-regulation also lays the groundwork for meaningful social communication in another way: it establishes a joint focus of communication between communication partners.

To explain this well, I need to back up a little bit, put on my speech language pathologist hat, and talk about the different types of communication. This is important to understand if we want kids to develop competence as communication partners within increasingly complex and meaningful exchanges. When kids start to communicate, they first do so to request and protest. Think about when kids are young; they communicate when they are hungry, tired, want something that they can't reach, etc. They also become good at letting us know what they don't want and communicating when they need comforting, for example when they are hurt. These are all important communicative functions (reasons to communicate).

But, as we become social beings, and develop deeper relationships, we go beyond requesting and protesting, or beyond communication that meets our personal needs. We begin to communicate for purely social purposes. For example, we communicate around external ideas, events, objects in our environment, memories, and plans. When we communicate about something separate from ourselves, that may be of mutual interest to another person (our communication partner), this is called joint attention. We (ourselves and our communication partner) are jointly attending to something other than ourselves, at the same time, and communicating to share observations and ideas around this separate thing.

An early example of joint attention is when we observe a toddler hear an airplane in the sky, point to it, and then look to their caregiver to share that point of interest. You don't need words to communicate for joint attention, you just need the ability to focus on something of interest, outside of yourself, and direct your communication partner's attention to it. Of course, this only gets more complex and deeper as we grow in our communication skills and language. For example, whereas a toddler may communicate by pointing out the airplane, an older child may be able to exchange memories with another person about a time when they were on a plane. Joint attention starts in the here and now, but then expands to include sharing memories and thinking about the future. It is important!

Kids with social learning differences are often first identified because this important area of development (communicating for joint attention) may not be as developed as expected. Or they may be skilled at requesting and protesting, but less so when it comes to communicating about a topic of mutual interest.

Here is the great news about co-regulation. It helps kids and their communication partners actively establish and maintain a joint focus of attention. It gives kids and their communication partners practice being in sync as they attend to an external event, object, or idea. Co-regulation lays the groundwork for joint attention between communication partners because it helps establish a shared focus. It gives everyone practice sustaining attention to the same idea over time, and it develops and unfolds into meaningful communication naturally. And because co-regulation keeps two individuals in sync, it also gives parents and caregivers practice knowing how to best support their child in the moment. It helps both caregivers and kids get connected to each other and stay connected! Awesome, right?

Co-regulation lays the groundwork for joint attention between communication partners because it helps establish a shared focus. It gives everyone practice sustaining attention to the same idea over time, and it develops and unfolds into meaningful communication naturally.

So now you might be wondering… how does this happen on a technical or practical level?

Co-regulation starts by giving everyone the opportunity to coordinate actions. The coordinating of actions helps establish a reciprocal flow between communication partners—I go/You go… I go/You go. This is what conversation is essentially—I say something/You say something…I respond/You respond…. I share an idea/You share an idea…etc.

When we create co-regulatory patterns that allow kids practice engaging in the reciprocal nature of communication, without placing language demands on them, we are laying the groundwork for them to internalize the reciprocal nature of conversation. We start by coordination actions. Sometimes this may be collaborative in nature, for example around a shared goal, or the goal may be simply to have fun or be present in the moment with that other person.

So that I do not stay too abstract, here are some examples across both types of ideas:

Co-regulation where we are present in the moment with the other person and have no specific end goal:

Playing catch – Imagine tossing a ball back and forth. You could be close or far away. It might be a basketball, or a baseball and you are wearing mitts. Or it may be with a toddler and you are rolling the ball back and forth on the floor. No matter what you are using or how you are delivering the ball, you share roles of "sender" and "receiver," and you need each other to keep the game going.

Playing Peekaboo – This is an in the moment activity that usually brings shared laughter. Contingent roles are "hider" and "finder." Imagine a caregiver covering her face with her hand, and then the baby pulls the caregiver's hands away so that they see each other again. The game is contingent because each person is needed, and the only goal is a joyful exchange together.

Light off/Light on – Here is an example that I often show on video of my sons when they were little. It always makes me laugh! In the clip, Freddie is age 3 and Desmond is around 18 months old. Desmond is in his crib and Freddie darts over to the light switch next to the crib and turns it off. There is silence in the darkness, as Freddie sits quietly on the floor. Moments later, Desmond turns on the light with a big laugh and shrieks with delight. He had crawled over to the light switch, pulled himself to stand, and proudly turned on the light. Once the light is on, he falls back onto his mattress. Freddie laughs wildly too and darts to the light switch again, turning it off once more. Again, silence in the darkness as both boys remain quiet. A few moments pass and Desmond turns on the light again, this time with an even bigger laugh and shriek! Freddie darts to turn off the light again, and the game continues. This was one of the first times I saw the boys really engage in co-regulation on their own, and observed how much joy it brought to them to engage in this reciprocal exchange where they had different roles, but each boy was competent in their own. It was balanced, fun for both, and they could continue it on their own without my help.

Now, examples of co-regulation that move toward a collaborative goal:

Group mural – I have another video clip that I love to share of two 7-year-old children, Anna and David. I taped a big piece of paper on the wall and suggested that we make a group mural. We could draw any scene together—for example, a city, a jungle, or a zoo. Anna and David chose a city. I created a co-regulatory pattern and competent roles by saying they would each take turns adding one thing. When you were the "draw-er," you could choose your marker color and add an idea. When you were not drawing, you were the "watcher," sitting close by and observing your peer add an item. What was beautiful to see was that, as they got going, they began to add items that were related to each other. Anna added a building, and David added some clouds in the sky. David added a sidewalk, then Anna added people walking on it. They added contingent ideas spontaneously, which was made possible by their contingent roles (or the co-regulatory pattern). I was able to sit back quietly and let them continue with the pattern and sharing of ideas. Then, amazingly, deeper conversation evolved as they used this joint focus of attention and shared goal (drawing a city) to talk about their family. After Anna drew people walking, she said, "This can be my Grandma." David then asked, "What about your Grandpa?" to which Anna responded, "My

Grandpa died last year," and a conversation in which they learned more about each other, unfolded. I could not have prompted this beautiful, touching conversation in the same way. It evolved spontaneously, around their joint focus of attention and ideas, and naturally created this opportunity for them to get to know each other and share of themselves. They shared of themselves and communicated curiosity about each other, but it was the co-regulatory activity, and the coordinating of actions that created the space for this to develop naturally. It still moves me to think of this exchange and watch this video clip.

They added contingent ideas spontaneously, which was made possible by their contingent roles, or the co-regulatory pattern. I was able to sit back quietly and let them continue with the pattern and sharing of ideas. Then, amazingly, deeper conversation evolved as they used this joint focus of attention and shared goal to talk about their family.

Sweeping together – I have another video clip I love to share of Eliza and her mother sweeping. I mentioned this in Chapter 2 as well. They worked together around Christmas time to sweep pine needles off the floor. Initially, Eliza was the "dustpan-holder" and her mother was the "sweeper." Then, they swapped roles once Eliza's mother knew her daughter would be competent in sweeping, having observed how she did it.

Grocery store – In my video clip of Nick (age 7) and his mother, Sue, Nick's role was to push the grocery cart, while Sue's role was to read the grocery list and point out needed items on the shelf. As she did so, Nick's role expanded to be the "getter" and he took items off the shelf and placed them in the cart. A grocery store can be a busy place and focusing on the same thing at the same time

30

could be a challenge for Sue and Nick. However, providing Nick a competent role that was contingent on Sue's role in this way allowed them to stay present to their shared task moment-to-moment over the course of the trip. Similarly, when they got to the car with their groceries, he was the "hander" and she was the "placer" as they put them in the back of the car. Even this aspect of the routine became a sweet, positive exchange that could not have happened if Sue did all the work herself while Nick sat in the back of the car. Conversationally, throughout this trip to the store, Nick and Sue were able to talk about their list together, remember what they needed, and plan for meals in the upcoming week. And, because he was authentically included in the process of shopping, they formed memories together which they could then later talk about and Nick could learn from. Remember that seeing moments through the lens of co-regulation allows you to notice and create authentic social exchanges that you can later build upon!

Seeing moments through the lens of co-regulation allows you to notice and create authentic social exchanges that you can later build upon.

Shredding paper - You may also remember Christopher and his mother, Judy, from Chapter 2 and *Declarative Language Handbook*. Judy engaged Christopher, age 21 at the time, in shredding paper. She had the role of "hander" and he had the role of "shredder." They stayed connected moment-to-moment as she handed him piles of paper, he commented on his role, learned a new job, and helped his mom out. Remember, things that you think you need to get done on your own when you have time, are often the best opportunities to create co-regulation and authentic connections and memories.

Things that you think you need to get done on your own when you have time, are often the best opportunities to create co-regulation and authentic connections and memories.

Shoveling snow – Here is another story! You may remember Gary and Jack from "Chapter 6: Making Mistakes is Okay" in *Declarative Language Handbook*. In this example of co-regulation, Gary invited Jack to help him shovel the driveway after a snowstorm. Gary was touched in how they worked in collaboration to break up the ice and then shovel it away. Gary was the "chopper," using an ice pick, while Jack was the "shoveler," scooping up and tossing the ice to the side. They coordinated actions moment-to-moment as they cleared their driveway, staying together in thought and conversation about the job at hand. And as with each of these examples, they also created a shared memory to reflect on and talk about later.

As each set of partners engaged in these opportunities, coordinating actions moment-to-moment, they slowed down to stay in tune with each other, and to better read each other's communicative cues as a result. What evolved was conversation and exchanges around their shared experiences. Jack and his dad talk about the ice and the driveway. Anna and David begin to talk about taking a walk in a city, and their grandparents. Freddie and Desmond, though not talking yet, share laughter together and form a meaningful memory. (That we still laugh about today!) Nick and his mom may begin to think about their next trip to the grocery store. Judy and Christopher stay connected as they talk through a task that could lead to meaningful employment.

In fact, each of these experiences lays the groundwork for future conversation in addition to conversation in the moment. Because you are slowing down and staying together moment-to-moment through each of these experiences, you are forming memories together that will later feed forward to conversation (i.e. *Remember that time we shoveled the driveway? That was hard work, but we did it!*). It also supports the child to remember and share these experiences with others as opportunities arise (e.g. Jack may hear someone else talking about shoveling snow and he could then chime in, "I shoveled with my Dad last weekend!").

So, although co-regulation may seem simple in the moment or slow when you get started, it serves so many important communication and social purposes. First and foremost, it gives everyone practice maintaining a joint focus of attention over time. In today's distracted world, I find this to be especially important. It teaches us how to be present to each other, gives us space to enjoy the here and now as we assume meaningful roles with each other, and deepens our relationships and memories with each other by letting us truly feel connected.

In today's distracted world, this is especially important: Co-regulation teaches us how to be present to each other, gives us space to enjoy the here and now as we assume meaningful roles with each other, and deepens our relationships and memories with each other by letting us truly feel connected.

CHAPTER 5:

Moving Towards Independence: Co-Regulation and Executive Function

As with the chapter on self-regulation, I'd like to define executive function in my own words, as I think about it, and as I take meaning from it in relation to kids with social learning differences. There are many exceptional books and materials out there on executive function—for example the work of Sarah Ward and Kristen Jacobsen at Cognitive Connections and *Smart but Scattered* by Peg Dawson and Richard Guare. If you want to dive deep into the area of executive function, those are the places to go. But, for our purposes, here it is defined in my own words...

Executive function is the process through which we first conceive an idea; picture what the end product looks like, and think through both the steps we may need to take to get it done as well as the materials we may need. Then, get started (initiate), sustain attention to the task for as long as needed, manage distractions along the way—both internal (I have to go to the bathroom!) and external (what's my brother doing?)—in order to shift our attention back to the task as needed. And last, stick with it (persist) until we are done. That is a lot, but we are still not done! Enveloping all these pieces is time management. We need to have a sense of whether we can complete the task in the time we have available, or whether we may need to plan to do it a different day, and/or do the task in smaller chunks over the course of time. Phew!

Executive functioning is a complex process and it's amazing that it all comes together seamlessly for many of us. Importantly, executive function skills develop as kids grow, and to be an independent and successful social being in life, you need to have solid executive functioning skills. And, executive function in adulthood translates to employment, relationships (e.g. following through on plans made with another person), and living on your own (getting the many tasks of daily living done, such as laundry, cooking, cleaning, shopping, hygiene, etc.). When young, kids need to use their developing executive function skills to do things like clean their room from start to finish, complete their homework on time, and even carry out the steps within an imaginative play scheme. Executive functioning skills are incredibly important, yet we know how hard these can be for kids with social learning differences.

Executive functioning skills are incredibly important, yet we know how hard these can be for kids with social learning differences.

Okay... so here is where co-regulation comes in. If kids are not yet independent in their ability to follow through with any task that has more than one step, how do we help them get there? One common practice might be to prompt each step using imperative language—*do this, okay now do that.* (Refer to *Declarative Language Handbook* for more about imperative language.) That may get the task done, but it does not help the child become independent if we are constantly prompting. Sometimes I have seen people use a visual checklist of steps that the child can refer to, to move themselves along and do what is needed. I think a checklist is great if the child can independently reference it and keep themselves on track. But, if an adult must continually prompt the child to attend to the checklist, then we are back where we started—prompting each step—unless they are remembering more of the steps on their own over time. Watch the child's feedback in the moment to determine if they are internalizing the steps, which allows you to fade back over time, or if you are both stuck.

Now I want to talk about a different way (a better way in my opinion) that does not rely on the constant step-by-step prompting described above. With co-regulation, you embrace a completely different mindset. You are not pushing the child to be independent one step at a time (*push, push, push...do this, okay now do that...*), you are instead engaging them as a partner in the process of doing XYZ, assigning them competent roles along the way, and gradually transferring responsibility as you see they are ready and can handle it. You are sharing the work, watching their feedback in the moment, pacing yourself and keeping them successful. In RDI, we often talk about this process as the master/apprentice relationship. You are someone who knows more (the master) and you are gradually giving the child (your apprentice), responsibility as they are ready. Your goal is always to transfer all responsibility over time (independence), but you know that is not where you start.

Your goal is always to transfer all responsibility over time (independence), but you know that is not where you start.

When we engage kids in multistep tasks with this mindset, everything shifts. It becomes a positive interaction rather than a negative, prompted one, and we both own the learning. We are able to thoughtfully consider what may be successful for the child and adjust as they are ready for more. The communication remains positive because we are using declarative language and because we approach the situation as a team. Everything can feel better when we do it from a place of sincere togetherness.

When we engage kids in multistep tasks with this mindset, everything shifts. It becomes a positive interaction rather than a negative, prompted one, and we both own the learning. We are able to thoughtfully consider what may be successful to the child and adjust as they are ready for more.

Here are some examples to help make this concrete for you:

Recently my boys had to clean their room. We hadn't cleaned in a while and things had really gotten out of hand. Through my lens, I could see so many things that needed to get done: clothes in the hamper, clean laundry put away, change their bedsheets, books on the bookshelf, wrappers and broken toys cleaned off the floor, get rid of things we don't use anymore, match socks in their overflowing sock drawer. Believe me, it went on and on. But, if I just said to them, *Clean your room!* they would have picked things up off the floor, put them on their bed or maybe thrown clothes in their hamper, and concluded they were done.

This was a much bigger task. I knew they could not see all that I saw because they are 8 and 11, and their vision and experiences thus far are different from mine. Although I may not have wanted to spend the afternoon cleaning, I knew the best way to get the job done was to do it in partnership with them and assign them competent roles as we moved along. Competent roles for the boys starting out included taking sheets off their bed and putting clothes in the hamper. They could do these things independently. Then, putting clean sheets on their beds required a tighter partnership with me and guidance using declarative language. My goal was to transfer my knowledge to them, so that someday soon they may be able to this job their own.

Declarative language to guide and establish these partnerships sounded like this: *Hmmm...Let's see what way the sheet goes. The short side goes along this way...Okay you can get the top and I'll get the bottom.* We needed to work together and coordinate our actions to complete the task. Yes, I could've done it on my own a lot quicker, but my goal is for these boys is to be independent young men who are capable and willing to help out around the house.

Then, there were many (many!) books on the floor! When left to their own devices, they tossed the books messily on the shelf every which way. Using declarative language, I helped them think ahead like I could: *If we place them like that, they are just going to fall and we have to pick them up again.* And then I guided them, in partnership, to do it well the first time. *Tell you what...How about if you hand me the books, one at a time, and I'll show you how to arrange them so they are neat, so we can see each of them, and so they don't all fall to the floor the minute we walk away.* Those are just two of the examples where I used co-regulation that day.

Another example where you can start to engage your child in activities of daily living, using co-regulation and partnership, is laundry! Even a 3-year-old could be part of this, if you define a competent role. Maybe the child could hand you an item, and you put it in the washing machine. Or maybe a preschooler could help you sort clothes into light and dark piles. You may be the one to set up the piles, and be the "hander" but then you can guide your child as to where each item may go, using declarative language to help them learn the process: *Hmmm...This shirt is white, so I'll hand it to you and you can put it with the lighter clothes. Here's the next one. It is dark blue...Let's put it in the dark pile. I'll hand it to you, and you can put it in this pile.* As you go, the child may need more guidance and support at the beginning, but imagine once they have learned the pattern and process, and how you could then fade back from guiding them with language, to simply handing them an item and then they visually scan and decide which pile to put it in.

It is these simple daily tasks that have so many learning opportunities embedded in them. Once you change your mindset and understand the partnership of co-regulation, you can make even the most mundane chore an opportunity for learning and social connection, while working towards independence in life!

You may wonder how this develops or becomes more sophisticated as kids grow. Picture this…It may start with your child sorting clothes by color, because that is a competent role for them, but once they've got that done, you can then introduce them to more steps—for example, what happens after you sort? Or before you sort what do you need to do to get ready? When you can see the big picture in this way, the potential and possibilities for learning keep growing. The sky is the limit when you approach things from a competent role perspective and engage in a positive manner of partnership and co-regulation. You are working towards independence in a positive way, long before you really need to think about it.

And here is the other cool thing. When you start from a place of competence, kids feel when they have mastered something and they often seek out the next challenge on their own. So, maybe sorting clothes by color when you hand an item one at a time has become easy. The child will be ready and willing for more responsibility and may initiate expanding their role. This is the beauty of co-regulation and competent roles—the child asks for more! This does not happen when we are prompting and prodding and pushing each step. With co-regulation, the child feels empowered to take on more, because the first part of the task has become easy for them. This is the nature of human growth—after we experience mastery in something, we are usually ready for the next challenge. We want kids to experience this feeling of mastery so that they can then seek the next manageable challenge and be an active member in their own learning journey.

When you start from a place of competence, kids feel when they have mastered something and they often seek out the next challenge on their own.

Here is an example related to an older child. I worked with an older teen, George, and his parents. Using these ideas, they helped him become independent in preparing his own meals. They started with one meal that they knew he enjoyed and within which they could create competent roles for him—making scrambled eggs. His mom, Carly, was alongside him for a while in the beginning—helping him think through ingredients, and giving him competent roles. For example, at first cracking eggs was not a competent role, so she did that, but stirring the eggs and pouring them into the pan were. So, George stirred and poured, but over time he practiced and became competent in cracking eggs and cooking, too. Appraising when the eggs were done was also tricky at first. But alongside each other, with George as Carly's apprentice, she guided him using declarative language as to what to notice and how to decide when they were cooked enough. (e.g. *I think when the eggs are fluffy and you can see the bottom of the pan with no liquid, the eggs are cooked enough.*) Carly took her time teaching him each of these processes, in partnership and using competent roles. As George became competent, she transferred more and more responsibility to him. George now makes several of his own meals and helps with meal planning. His parents are now helping him become proficient in making a grocery list and looking for coupons! But his parents and I will always remember that it started with scrambled eggs.

Chapter 5: Moving Towards Independence

So here is what I want you to remember. You can start working on executive functioning skills and eventual independent living anytime you want. Use co-regulation and a mindset of partnership to guide your child through new opportunities or effortful tasks, by assigning them competent roles along the way. Your mindset is not: *do this, do that, get that done...* This approach will make everyone frustrated. Rather, your mindset is: I have knowledge and skills, and I will transfer these to you as your partner and at a pace that keeps you successful. We start where we start. We are in this together, and who knows... maybe we will even have fun!

PART 3:

MECHANICS

CHAPTER 6:

Frameworks and Declarative Language: How to "Do" Co-Regulation

Here we go! The nuts and bolts of co-regulation. I discussed some of this in Chapter 2. In this chapter, I will repeat what is important but then get a bit more into examples and the logistics of creating co-regulatory opportunities with kids. I would like to give credit to Dr. Steven Gutstein, Dr. Rachelle Sheely, and the RDI Community of both former and current RDI Consultants for the ideas I am about to express. Everything I understand and know about co-regulation was taught to me within this community. As a group of professionals, we understand co-regulation well, and are constantly further guiding each other's learning and providing examples on how to incorporate these ideas into our work in meaningful ways. If you want to understand co-regulation beyond this book, the RDI community is a great place to go!

Now onto what I can teach you in this book.

First, the basics. Remember, as you engage in co-regulation you are thinking about creating partnerships, and partnerships within everyday moments and daily routines are the best because this is what will help us engage kids in these ways frequently, because we have to do XYZ anyway! These opportunities are also what will help our kids learn and grow because we are using naturally occurring, everyday moments that are meaningful and real.

These opportunities are also what will help our kids learn and grow because we are using naturally occurring, everyday moments that are meaningful and real.

Start by approaching a task or process that you may typically do on your own, or that may typically be a one-person job. Think about how you could carve this process into a two-person job, where both people have a role that is authentic and contingent on the other person's, while always ensuring the child has a role in which they can be competent—competent, authentic, contingent roles. This is what we talked about in Chapter 2.

Now for the new stuff... How do you find or create these types of roles across different activities, in an ongoing way? In RDI, we like to think of different frameworks, or ways to create roles with different frameworks in mind. Here are the main ones, and I think once you conceptualize these, you will start to see opportunities for roles in a variety of different places. I have included a description of the framework, along with real examples that I have seen in my work with kids and families. I will list them here and then expand on each one below:

1. Assembly Line
2. Complementary
3. Parallel
4. Reciprocal

Chapter 6: Frameworks and Declarative Language

1. **Assembly Line** – in other words: you – me – place.

   Examples:
   a. *Cleaning up toys* - I hand you a toy, and you put it in its place.
   b. *Putting books on a bookshelf* - You hand me a book that is on the floor, I put it on the shelf, and then we start again.
   c. *In line at the grocery store* - You hand me an item, I put it on the conveyor belt, and so on.
   d. *Setting the table* - I hand you a plate, you put it on the table, and then I hand you the next one, and so on.
   e. *Doing laundry together* - I fold an item and hand it to you so you can put it in its place.

Get the gist? This one is easy and applicable in many different contexts once you are looking for it.

2. **Complementary** – This just means that my role complements yours, or my role adds to yours in a slightly different way. Our roles are different actions that are connected to each other.

   Examples:
   a. *We are sweeping together* - you are sweeping and I am holding the dustpan.
   b. *We are baking together* - you are holding the bowl while I stir the batter.
   c. *We are putting a pizza in the oven* - you open the oven door and I put in the pizza.
   d. *We are pouring milk* - you are holding the cup while I pour the milk.

e.   *We are unlocking a door* - I will put the key in and turn it, and you open the door.

f.   *We are making blueberry pancakes* - I am stirring and you are adding blueberries.

g.   *We are hanging up decorations* - you hold the decoration in place and I tape it.

h.   *We are cutting paper* - I hold the paper while you cut with scissors.

This one is fun, and again opportunities are everywhere once you start looking.

3. **Parallel** – We are doing the same thing at the same time, alongside each other. This is one of my favorites!

    Examples:
    a.   *We are carrying a recycling bin to the curb together* - you take one end and I take the other.

    b.   *We are carrying a laundry basket of clean clothes together* - you take one side and I'll take the other.

    c.   *We are walking together with your bike* - you take one handlebar and I take the other.

    d.   *We are walking the dog together* - both of us are holding the leash.

    e.   *We just cut down a Christmas tree and are carrying it together to the car* - you have the top and I have the bottom.

4. **Reciprocal** – I take a turn and then you take the same turn.

    Examples:

a. *We are making pizza* - I add a topping and then you add a topping.
b. *We are playing a board game* - I take my turn and then you take your turn.
c. *We are putting books on a shelf* - I place one book and then you place one book.
d. *We are adding items to our grocery list* - I write down one item, and then you write down the next item, and so on.

Using declarative language to name roles is what helps partnerships, social opportunities, and connections become visible and inviting to our kids with social learning differences.

As you create these roles, the next important element to keep in mind, the element that will help it all come together for kids, is to use *declarative language* to name the roles. This is what helps partnerships, social opportunities, and connections become visible and inviting to our kids with social learning differences. Often, through natural interactions many kids and adults find ways to come together and work together without saying much. We read the context and each other, and find a way in. But this is what can be hard for kids with social learning differences. They are unsure how to enter an exchange or activity, so they may stay on the periphery and not join at all. As you use declarative language to name and narrate how to be together, you make this very elusive process concrete, which helps them feel comfortable joining. It will also help them know how to join similar social contexts in the future. Here are some example declarative statements that go with the opportunities listed previously where you are naming each person's role and actions:

I'll hand you the books one at a time and you can put them on the shelf.
I'll take this side of the laundry basket and you can take that side.
I can help. Let's pull your bike back to the garage together. I'll take this handlebar and you can take that one.
You can hold the dustpan while I sweep.

You can also name the roles using a label ending in "-er". Examples:

I'll be the dish hander, and you can be the dish placer.
We can be recycling bin carriers together.
You can be the bowl holder and I'll be the stirrer.
Let's take turns being ingredient adders.

There is something wonderful about naming a role. Kids rise to own it. What has also been wonderful to see in my experience, is that as we start to use this language with kids, they then spontaneously start to use it with others as a purposeful way to navigate social interactions in partnership. They simply needed the knowledge of a framework and possible language to use, along with concrete strategies, to feel empowered joining and staying connected over time.

As you engage kids in different processes, remember that you can be flexible. Their role does not need to stay the exact same throughout the entire process of what you are doing together. In fact, you may opt to change roles, swap roles, or create new roles with a different framework within the context of the same process. This is all good and a way to keep a process moving forward, fluidly, in a positive way. The most important thing to keep in mind is that you make sure the child remains competent in the new role you are creating. You will likely know when they are no longer competent because you are prompting more, or they have become bored and seem less engaged which indicates it is too easy.

As the "master" and guide, it is your job to read the child's feedback in the moment and make adjustments to keep what they are doing at the "just right" level of challenge for them (not too easy, not too hard). You may also transfer responsibility as you go (as we talked about in Chapter 5) so that their role grows over time. I will discuss this idea more in the next chapter.

Remember too, as you engage in these types of co-regulatory opportunities, you are also going to be thinking about your pace to ensure that you stay together with the child as you move through the process of what you are doing. You need to be a team, which means if one person is not doing their job, then it does not get done. As with declarative language, pacing is extremely important. So important in fact, that it gets its own chapter. Stay tuned... that topic will be coming up in Chapter 8.

CHAPTER 7:
Adjusting Complexity

Next, we will discuss the fluidity of co-regulation and managing its ups and downs. Practicing this idea may seem easiest when kids are young, but I want you to know that co-regulation is not only for young kids. If you are wearing your competent roles mindset, you can scale what you are doing up or down, depending on the child. What you are always going for is the sweet spot between where your child is bored because something is too easy, and where your child is overwhelmed because something is too hard. This is called their "edge of competence" and it is constantly moving as a child grows and learns in the company of others. This idea was first introduced by Russian psychologist Lev Vygotsky who defined it using the term "zone of proximal development."

What you are always going for is the sweet spot between where your child is bored because something is too easy, and where your child is overwhelmed because something is too hard. This is called their "edge of competence" and it is constantly moving as a child grows and learns in the company of others.

That means that for a younger child, you may need to create a role that has few materials, few actions to do, or few decisions to make, in order to ensure they are competent. But, for a teenager, this may mean that you can zoom out to engage them as your partner in a more sophisticated learning opportunity where they have multiple opportunities to make decisions, need to shift their attention between ideas and materials more frequently, or may even need to include multiple people in the process of what they are doing. A concrete example of this is teaching a teenager to drive. Think about all the elements a person needs to consider once they are behind the wheel!

As we add or scale back elements, we are thinking about "complexity." And, regardless of the complexity of what you are doing together, with co-regulation you are always there as the child's partner and guide, showing them the way with love, support, and positive communication.

The main elements of any process or activity that adds complexity and over which you have control are: your space, your physical proximity, the materials you are using, the decision-making opportunities within the activity, your language, and the number of people involved. We will go through each one below, and your first step will be to consider these prior to inviting your child to an activity, because you want to set yourselves up for success (both you *and* your child!). Remember, these are all moving parts that you can scale up, or scale down, depending on whether your child needs more or less of a challenge. Here we go:

1. **Your space** – At any given time, you can think about where you are. Are you inside? Outside? Are you at a store, or at home? Then, what does the space you are working at look like? A cleared off table? On the floor with toys surrounding you? Are devices such as phones or tablets nearby or put off to the side and on silent?

Your space can be unintentionally distracting, or it can create positive challenges related to attention. You get to decide what your child needs to be successful and at their edge of competence. A younger child may need you to be close and in a space that is clear of distractions. Your teenager may need you to have them put their phone away before starting. Does a busy environment cause a power struggle? (For example, they keep playing with a toy and you keep asking them to put it down or put it away.) Or is your child getting competent at independently filtering out distractions in the environment that are not important in the here and now? Know that you have control over your space and what you want it to look like before engaging your child in something new. Set your child up for success by adjusting your space accordingly. Example: if they can't yet *"not"* be distracted by the toy on the table while you are trying to do something together, put the toy somewhere else before you get started.

2. **Physical proximity** – How close are you to each other?

Sometimes kids need us right next to them or across from them, but sometimes we can stand back and observe while they move through something that they have learned. Know that your location is a variable you can make thoughtful, moment-to-moment decisions about as you support your child. For example, do they need you close by to support attention and help them remember their role? Or can they sustain their attention and manage distractions with you a little further back?

Here is a concrete example of this idea in practice: when doing math homework, your child may need you to sit alongside them as they practice a new concept, but as they learn and master the concept, you can probably get up and walk away, only coming back to check in periodically.

Your child needs you closer or further away depending on the level of challenge that they face. This is okay! Keep in mind your physical position can be fluid as you adjust based on their needs in the moment.

3. **Materials** – How many items are you actively using at one time?

Starting out, fewer materials are best. This is because you first want co-regulation to be about you and the child. As you have more things, they can get in the way of your connection to your child. More materials can mean more distraction. So beginning co-regulation activities will have less materials. For example: you may hand a book one at a time to your child as they put them on the shelf or you may carry one bag together, each taking a handle.

However, as your child grows, and as they can successfully shift their attention between materials and you, and the task at hand, you can thoughtfully include more materials, or choose activities that have more materials by nature. If we think about the bookshelf example, starting out you are close and handing a book one at a time. But as you add complexity in terms of materials, maybe you hand two at a time. Or you may leave some of the floor and let the child choose which one is next, knowing they will not get too distracted by all the choices.

Here is another example while working together in the kitchen: initially, you may simply hand your child an ingredient to put in a bowl to make something to eat – for example, a fruit salad. You are close with few materials on the table in the child's line of sight. But, as your child grows in their competence, you engage them as your partner in more complex recipes that require several ingredients. Early on within the more complex recipe, you may support their attention by having only one ingredient in sight at a time, but as your child's attentional capacity grows, you may have all of them out on the table.

You are basing the number of materials in sight and in your working space on your child's attentional success and then adding in elements as you notice they can handle it. You are watching to see how your child successfully shifts attention between materials, the process of what you are doing, and you. Can they do it independently or do they become distracted? You can modify this at any time if you notice the challenge is too great, or not great enough.

You will know the challenge is too great if you are finding yourself involved in power struggles about what your child is looking at or trying to hold. If you hear yourself saying, *Pay attention!* again and again, chances are there are too many materials and it will help both of you if you move some things to the side. Don't hesitate to do this, because setting the scene up for your child's success proactively feels a lot better than prompting them constantly to pay attention.

If you hear yourself saying, *Pay attention!* again and again, chances are there are too many materials and it will help both of you if you move some things to the side. Don't hesitate to do this, because setting the scene up for your child's success proactively feels a lot better than prompting them constantly to pay attention.

Remember too… These ideas are fluid and attention will grow! Just because you are scaling back now does not mean you will never be able to do an activity with multiple materials. Rather, it means you are getting there slowly and steadily, at a pace your child can manage and at a pace that keeps them competent. You are building their attentional capacity a little at a time, and along the way helping them know what is important to attend to.

4. **Decision-making opportunities** - In any activity or process that you do, there are moment-to-moment decisions that need to be made. For example, in what order do you do things? What do you need to do next? How much, how long, how far, how hard, etc. should you do something? How much time should you spend on something and when is it time to move on? "Appraisal" is another word for these fluid, moment-to-moment judgements that can be big or small. We are constantly making appraisals in life about everything we do. In fact, we do it so much that we often don't even think about it!

"Appraisal" is another word for these fluid, moment-to-moment judgements that can be big or small.

As you engage your child in both beginning and then more complex activities, start to notice the decisions you make. It is exciting to realize that this is also an element that you can transfer responsibility as your child is ready. To go back to the bookshelf example, initially you may be making the decision around which book to place next or where to place each one. But, as your child gains competence, these are probably decision-making opportunities you can offer them. Or when cooking, you guide your child to follow a recipe in terms of how much salt to add, but perhaps a decision you can gradually transfer to them as they gain competence is, *Do you think that is enough salt? Let's taste it and see.* Here is another example: when grocery shopping, perhaps you can offer your child the decision of what section of the grocery store to start in, while also guiding them to realize it is probably best to do frozen foods towards the end of your trip!

As you engage your child in both beginning and then more complex activities, start to notice the decisions you make. It is exciting to realize that this is also an element that you can transfer responsibility as your child is ready.

Decision-making is a fun area to explore and think about, because there are likely so many decisions you make for your child. But as you support them to grow into increasingly independent adults, you can think about where you would like to fade back and give them opportunity to make small decisions, while benefiting from your thoughtful assurance along the way.

5. **Language** – Think about what you are saying! Are you talking in sentences? Single words or simple word combinations? Are you communicating abstract ideas? Is your vocabulary related primarily to the here and now (your current space and activity)? Or are you recalling memories or thinking about future plans that are helpful to consider in this moment?

   When considering your language, also consider your child's current language level. Adjust your language complexity to match your child's developmental level. If they are an emerging language user, or not yet talking, you can keep your language to single words or simple phrases, or even intonation patterns, and use rich nonverbal communication to support their comprehension. But, if your child is older and talkative, and has comprehension to match, then your language can be more sophisticated too.

When considering your language, also consider your child's current language level. Adjust your language complexity to match your child's developmental level.

You may also want to consider your child's comprehension in terms of language abstraction. If they have a good handle on abstract language (language outside of the here and now, language that requires some nonliteral interpretation such as figurative language or making inferences), then feel free to talk abstractly about what you are teaching. But, if your child is a concrete language user, be mindful of this as you speak so that you keep them competent. You are welcome to use more abstract language as you make the conscious decision to increase complexity in this area. But know that it will be helpful and important to explain what you mean using declarative language, so they learn. For example, if time is tight and you say, *We have to shake a leg,* you are using abstract language. Follow up with, *That means we have to hurry,* so you are also teaching at the same time.

Another important aspect of language use is knowing when to talk and when to NOT talk. Often, it is important to be quiet so your child can think about what to do next. As you gain competence yourself in leading co-regulatory teaching opportunities, start to notice when it is important for you to use declarative language to guide or explain, and when it is more important for you to be quiet so your child can do the mental work that you are giving them the opportunity to do. Silence is an important and underrated tool! You can teach when you are quiet. Remember this! We will talk more about this in the next chapter on pacing.

Another important aspect of language use is knowing when to talk and when to NOT talk. Often, it is important to be quiet so your child can think about what to do next.

---

6. **Number of People** – How many people (kids or adults) are involved in what you are doing? Anytime we do something with our child, there might be other people around. But with co-regulation, it is always best to start with only you and your child. It is possible to create co-regulatory patterns with more than two people, but when first practicing and gaining competence in co-regulation, keep it simple so both you and your child can master the basics of *you* and *me* doing something together first.

When thinking about adding more people to what you are doing, I want you to consider this... As with materials and language, more is more. More people translates to: more actions to attend to, more language to process and respond to, and more varying intentions and agendas to be aware of. This can get challenging fast, which is why kids with social learning differences can experience conflict or setbacks with peers. It is hard work!

As you consider adding in more people to your co-regulatory patterns with your child, it is important to do so thoughtfully, and at a pace both you and your child can manage. If you want to add a sibling, for example, before you get started, consider what will be competent roles for *both* children. Or you may want to consider what framework will be most successful as you add another person. For example, when setting the table, you could use an assembly line pattern to work together (I hand you a cup, and you hand it to your brother, who then places it on the table) or a complementary pattern (You are in charge of plates, your sister is in charge of cups, and I am in charge of silverware). Or, maybe using a parallel pattern is just right (Let's all take hold of this side of the table as we push it together to move it where we want it to be).

As you consider adding in more people to your co-regulatory patterns with your child, it is important to do so thoughtfully, and at a pace both you and your child can manage.

In thinking about adding in another parent or caregiver to your co-regulation, it is critical that you work together. For example, if both parents are joining in a co-regulatory pattern with their child, be mindful not to talk at the same time or to perform actions at the same time in a way that competes for your child's attention. It is a wonderful thing when parents or caregivers can create co-regulatory patterns together with their child. But you must ensure that you are in sync and complementing each other, and not placing conflicting demands on your child.

In thinking about adding in another parent or caregiver to your co-regulation, it is critical that you work together. Ensure that you are in sync and complementing each other, and not placing conflicting demands on your child.

So, as you practice co-regulation and consider adding another person, set everyone up for success by thinking through competent roles for everyone within this new dynamic, and importantly, appreciate that doing something with only two people is very different than doing the same thing with three or more people. Add in more people at a pace that keeps your child successful.

I will also talk in more detail about peer interactions in Chapters 10 and 11. So, stay tuned for that!

Aside from these six elements, there is another way to expand an activity as your child is ready. You can expand an activity beyond what a child has mastered by including them in the steps *prior to* or *immediately after* what they have already learned. Within a grocery store routine, you may initially start by having your child help you put groceries away one at a time once you arrive home. However, once the child has mastered this, you could expand their role on the front end by including them in the process of creating your grocery list before you go shopping, and you could then invite them to help you reference the list while you are shopping. With this idea, you are including them in your thought processes and decision-making at the beginning, so that once you are at the store, they have a window into your plan and intended sequence of actions. These are ideas we talked about in Chapter 5 - Moving Towards Independence: Co-Regulation and Executive Function.

Here is another example of how to expand your child's role using this idea. Think about changing batteries in a toy or household item such as a flashlight. Initially, your child's role may be to hand you the batteries you need so you can put them in (assembly line), or maybe their role is to help you push the battery to lock it in place (parallel). But as they gain competence in these roles, you can offer new roles on the front end like deciding or discovering what size batteries are needed and then finding them in your house, and on the back end, such as what do you do with the old batteries once you replace them?

In summary, you have an important role to play as you transfer responsibility to your child! Imagine holding a rope that you gradually let out as your child is ready for more responsibility and independence, or that you gently pull back in as you realize you gave them too much. You consider and explore the elements discussed above as you transfer. *You* decide how to increase or decrease the challenge, depending on what will help your child remain competent. And because you know your child well, you are in the best position to make these decisions. You can add steps, take away steps, and include your child in decision-making opportunities that you feel they are ready for.

You **decide how to increase or decrease the challenge, depending on what will help your child remain competent. Because you know your child well, you are in the best position to make these decisions.**

Keep in mind that each of the elements discussed above will increase attentional demands as you add them and will give your child more to think about. So, add more as your child is ready. You always want to balance things so that your child is not bored and feels challenged, but is also not in over their head or overwhelmed. Competence is key. Add elements with your child's readiness and competence in mind - not all at once, but at a pace that keeps them positively engaged, eager to learn something new because they feel competent, and at that place that they will **succeed**.

PART 4:

PACING AND TROUBLESHOOTING

CHAPTER 8:

Using Pacing and Limit Setting to Create Balance

Just as pacing is extremely important when using declarative language (as discussed in *Declarative Language Handbook*), pacing is equally important as you practice co-regulation. You enter co-regulatory opportunities with the mindset of: *We are doing this together.* That means, at any given point, for whatever reason, if your child is not assuming their role, you need to pause what you are doing and wait.

With co-regulation, you are creating a rich feedback loop where you are reading your child's cues moment-to-moment to ensure (1) *they are competent*, (2) *they understand their role*, and (3) *they assume their role.* What helps make co-regulation most successful from the start is to actively name roles, as we discussed in Chapter 6. You may also need to not only name the role but describe it in language your child can understand. Or perhaps model what you mean if they are unsure. We will get into these tips more in Chapter 9. But with respect to pacing, as long as you are sure your child will be competent in their role, and you are sure they understand what it is they are supposed to do, then you must wait for them to assume their role when it is time for them to do so.

Here is an example. You comment, *Let's set the table. I'll hand you the plate, and you can put it on the table.* You then hold out a plate and wait. Wait for the child to notice, take it, and then place it. Do not over prompt or say the instruction again. Simply get in the habit of waiting quietly for the child to notice on their own that you are ready for them to do their part. Wait for them to shift their attention toward you, toward your outreached arm, to integrate all these pieces of information (i.e., your words, your gesture, the context), and then to assume their role. If you feel worried that they are not responding, a good rule of thumb starting out is to count to 30 in your head before you add more information. You want to give the child plenty of time to notice, process all the information, and be independent. If you prompt them too quickly, they are doing it because you prompted, not because they are authentically or independently assuming their role. Sometimes kids need help, and that is okay. We'll get into that in the next chapter. But first, I want you to practice waiting, so you get in the habit of giving them the time they may need to join the routine on their own.

With pacing, another important area that you are actively working on is the idea of breakdowns and repairs. You are giving the child time and space to observe when a breakdown, misunderstanding, or interruption of being sync, has happened, and then letting them be the ones to make the repair. This is a dynamic communication skill that is very important in life. Kids develop the ability to notice communication breakdowns early on in development. But if we are always fixing breakdowns for kids before they have a chance to notice on their own, we are not giving them the opportunity to develop this dynamic skill.

If we are always fixing communication breakdowns for kids before they have a chance to notice on their own, we are not giving them the opportunity to develop this dynamic skill.

Here is an example. Imagine you are playing catch. This is a nice co-regulatory pattern. I throw, you catch. Then you throw and I catch. It is reciprocal, it is balanced, and we certainly need each other to keep the game going. If at any point I miss the ball that you have thrown to me, you wait for me to retrieve it, pick it up, and toss it back to you to continue the game. This is a prototype of what happens with communication volleys. You send a message. I receive it. I send one back, and then you receive it. If at any point you don't receive what I have sent, then it is up to me or you to notice that we are no longer in sync. And one, or both of us, must make a repair.

For example, maybe you say, *I didn't get what you said. Can you say that again?* Or I say, *Hey! I think you didn't hear me. Let me say that again.* When you engage in a co-regulatory pattern, such as catch, and the child "misses" what we have sent (or we have missed what they have sent), fixing it for them does not help them better notice what they missed, or notice it has even happened. We must share this work with kids.

Here is how we do this. If we wait quietly upon noticing the breakdown, then the child is more likely to also notice that the breakdown has occurred. When we wait quietly, we allow them opportunity to notice that they have missed our message or perhaps that we have missed theirs, and they are more likely to work to repair this breakdown. For example, they may then send the message again, or send it in a different way. When using catch as an analogy for this idea, this might mean that the child runs to get the ball after noticing they missed it, picks it up, and then sends it back again for continued interactions.

As you pace yourself, or quietly wait for the child to assume their role, you are actively working on interactions being balanced, communicating to kids that they are needed, and helping them notice and make repairs. I can't emphasize enough how important waiting is. Interactions in life are meant to be balanced. We can make it so through co-regulatory opportunities.

As you pace yourself, or quietly wait for the child to assume their role, you are actively working on interactions being balanced and communicating to kids that they are needed.

Here is another example. Remember Judy and Christopher? I remember watching them carry a tote bag together as they walked down a hallway. It was beautiful! When Christopher let go of his handle and kept walking, Judy knew to stop in her tracks and wait quietly for Christopher to notice. Once he realized his mother was no longer with him, he stopped too. He turned to visually reference her to see what had happened, and she then guided his observations with a declarative statement: "You dropped your handle!" He then returned to her to make a repair (take the handle again) so they could continue together with the routine.

These moments are small and nuanced, but they are critical because they communicate to the child that they are a true partner. They communicate that the child is needed. They communicate that the child is important. As we pace and wait, and wait and observe, we help kids feel what it is like to be part of a balanced interaction. This is what communication is, and as you practice balance in these small moments of co-regulation, kids will internalize what a reciprocal, balanced exchange feels like. And you will too! The more you do it together, the easier it becomes. At times we may overcompensate for kids or over prompt, and pacing (pausing, watching, waiting quietly, as needed) should help you do this less.

There is another common type of imbalance within interactions as well: when the child tries to take over your role! Yes, this happens too. In some instances it may be a good thing, for example if you are working toward independence in a particular skill (i.e. if they are ready and willing to clean up their room on their own, let them do it!). But if you are working toward helping them share responsibility (i.e. if it is hard for the child to include others in a process) or if you are working to help the child be more open to the contributions of others, finding balance remains important.

The flip side of pacing is limit setting. Whereas with pacing you are slowing yourself down, with limit setting you are helping the child to pace and slow themselves down, so they remember to include you! To do this in the moment, you may set a limit or restate your roles using declarative language: *You just did X, but that was my job!*, and then wait for them to adjust their actions. For example, after you make the statement, they may pull their hand back, say, *Oh yeah! I forgot,* and leave space for you to join in again. An example of this would have been if Christopher took both handles of the bag he and Judy were carrying together. She could make the declarative statement, *Christopher, I wanted to hold one of the handles,* or *Christopher, I wanted to carry this bag together.* Next, she could wait quietly for him to let go of one handle, and she could take hold again, reestablishing their partnership and balance.

Whereas with pacing you are slowing yourself down, with limit setting you are helping the child to pace and slow themselves down, so they remember to include you!

This aspect of co-regulation practice helps kids scale back and share work with you in an ongoing way. It is important work to do, especially when kids are used to or most comfortable, doing things on their own. They may want to be in control of the entire task because that is most comfortable for them. Your goal in these instances is to help them feel more comfortable and at ease over time with sharing the work, so the exchange becomes balanced.

In summary, balance means you are both doing equal parts of the work. This may mean that you need to wait and pace yourself to allow the child time and space to assume their role, notice breakdowns, and make repairs. But it may also mean that you need to set limits and/or restate your contingent roles so that your child slows down to create space for you! Funny how it can work both ways with co-regulation, right?

What you do depends on your kids and whether at any moment in time, you are working to build their competence as your partner or working to build their comfort with sharing roles and responsibilities. Your means of establishing balance at any given time (slowing down or setting limits) will vary based on the routine you are doing together. For one activity, you may need to monitor your own pace, while for another you may need to help your child monitor theirs. But, as the master or guide to your child's apprentice, it is your job to decide. As you work to stay in sync with your child and keep in tune with their feedback moment-to-moment, it will become easier for you to know which to do.

CHAPTER 9:
Troubleshooting Tips

Just like in *Declarative Language Handbook,* this chapter will help
you think about what to do when your attempt to engage your
child in a co-regulatory pattern or activity does not work. When this
happens, do not be discouraged. There are things for you to consider
which will help you modify what you are doing in order to lead
to successful engagement. Here is how I think about and approach
breakdowns, or how I respond when my invitations or attempts at
engaging the child in co-regulation are not working.

First and foremost, I think to myself, *Is the role that I have assigned
the child the right role for them?* Quite often, the role is either too hard
or it is too easy, therefore they are not assuming their role in the way
I had intended.

**When something is not working, first and foremost, ask yourself, *Is
the role that I have assigned the child the right role for them?* Quite
often the role is either too hard or it is too easy.**

Other reasons might be because the child is unsure of their own
competence, or unsure of what is expected. When these are the
reasons, they often reveal themselves as a big "NO." The child may
feel some uncertainty or worry that is holding them back. When this

69

happens, it becomes my job to figure out exactly what the worry or uncertainty is, so we can problem solve through it.

I will go through each scenario, along with next steps.

First, step back and think about the role you have assigned the child.

1. *Might the child's role be too hard?* You can tell a role is too hard if you are prompting the child a lot to get them going—giving a lot of directions, perhaps thinking about using physical guidance or hand over hand assistance, or feeling like you need to push them along one step at a time to do their part. If the child cannot do what you are asking them to do on their own with just a tiny bit of help or guidance and time, then this is *not* a competent role. Think of a different role you could give them instead. Maybe the role needs to be a little smaller, a little less complex, or not take as long to complete.

   If you do feel confident that the role is competent, but you are not sure how to help the child be successful when they are stuck, then we will talk through some other ways to scaffold in the upcoming section. But first always ensure that the role is not too hard. That is the first step. Always!

2. *Is the role too easy?* Often when kids feel bored, they tune out and start to think about something else. Or they have trouble getting engaged because they may not feel a mental challenge. Yes, we all have to do the boring parts sometimes, but if your goal is sustained co-regulation to get to something greater, then you may want to think about how to increase the challenge for the child so that they have that spark in their heart and mind

that naturally engages them. To increase the challenge, refer to Chapter 7 and use tips and ideas about how to add complexity or transfer some of your responsibility to the child. They may be ready for it!

Next, is the child feeling unsure? If they are feeling worried or unsure of their own competence, you may want to troubleshoot by inviting them to share what they are thinking using declarative language. For example, you might say, *I'm wondering what you are thinking about this,* or *I'm trying to figure you why you don't want to do this right now.* Some kids might share with you what is getting in the way, and then you can problem solve or find ways to help them feel less worried.

If the child is feeling worried or unsure of their own competence, you may want to troubleshoot by inviting them to share what they are thinking using declarative language.

Scaffolding

Now, if you are sure that the role is not too hard or too easy, and you want to figure out how to help the child stay engaged as you expand or continue their role, you provide help by "scaffolding." I like this term better than the word "prompt" because it helps me visualize what we are trying to do.

When seen around a building, scaffolding is temporary. It is there to help as needed, and it is gradually taken down as the building stands on its own. This is what we want your support to be—temporary and dynamic. You add it as your child needs it, but you are watching their cues in the moment to determine how and when and in what manner to take it down, or gradually remove it. It may help to keep in mind the previously discussed idea of transferring responsibility to the child as you sense they are ready.

Here are examples of scaffolding, some of which interestingly, are like the supports described in *Declarative Language Handbook*, "Chapter 11: Troubleshooting Tips." Therefore, some of these ideas may be familiar but you now have a new context in which to consider them.

1. *Wait longer* – Sometimes we just need to wait a bit longer to let the child process what we have said or done. Count to 30 in your head, maintain the gesture you have assumed (e.g. if you are handing something to the child, continue to hold your hand out, giving them a chance to notice, process and respond, or if you are working to carry something together, pause next to that thing taking hold of one side, and wait for them to notice so they can take the other side).

2. *Use a guiding, declarative statement* - After you have waited a respectful amount of time and you feel the child has had enough time to process what you have said, and still has not responded, add a comment that provides either a reminder or more information about what you are doing together and what the child's role may be. Reminders can be declarative comments such as, *I'm waiting for you,* or *I can't do this without you,* or even *I'm wondering if you are ready yet.*

Additional information, if needed, might explain their role further or in a slightly different way so you know the child understands. Examples might be, *Okay, so when you are the sprayer, that means you spray a little of the cleaner on the table and then I will wipe*, or *When you are the dish placer, that means you put the plate, cup, or utensils in the dishwasher after I hand them to you*, or *When we are beach bag carriers together, that means I take one handle and you take the other*. Some kids really need this additional information as they learn new roles. Chances are once you have explained it and they have learned it, then they won't need the explanation again. But it can be important to slow down and provide this information in the beginning.

3. *Model -* Sometimes it can be helpful to model the action you are thinking or model the role you want the child to assume. The visual presentation can be especially important for visual learners. You can simply say something like this, *Here let me show you what I would do, and then you can give it a try*, or *I will go the first couple of times, and then when you are ready, you can go*. The idea of modeling can be especially helpful for older kids who are ready for more. Rather than modeling one step at a time, you may even consider modeling a few steps at a time if they are ready to take in more information at once. Remember, if you realize it is too much, you can always scale back and do less.

4. *Create a tighter partnership -* One enjoyable way to scaffold for kids is to partner with them more tightly within the specific role you have assigned. Yes, you were already partnering with them to start, but you may need to further break down and partner even within that first step that you had in mind for them. I find this especially helpful when kids are feeling worried or unsure as you engage them in something new. They might say

no to joining, so then I say something like, *That's okay. We can be partners, and both do your job until you feel ready to do it on your own.* As an example, this idea can be especially helpful in games with kids, where they are unsure of the rules or need additional support while they learn. I will talk more about this in the upcoming chapters on peer interaction too!

5. *Add a gesture -* Sometimes we may want to add a gesture that supports comprehension. For example, you may point or nod to something, or guide their attention to what they may not be noticing on their own. Example: imagine you are sweeping together, and the child does not see the crumbs that you do. To help them keep their role going of sweeper, you may say, *I see more crumbs over there!* while pointing. Or, when taking out the trash, you may guide with a point saying, *Oops! We dropped something right there. Let's pick that up.* Sometimes, a child just may need a little more help to understand what we are thinking.

6. *Use declarative language to help the child read the context -* We can always use declarative language to help kids decode a situation, or to explain the context at hand. We might know it intuitively, but they might not. Simply comment and explain at a level your child will understand. For example, *Hmm....I see some people up ahead. While we push this shopping cart, I think it will be a good idea to go slowly and move the cart around them.*

7. *Break down the role -* You can always go back to breaking their role down to a smaller role, and building it back up once you see they are ready and competent. Remember, this process is fluid, and you want to hold onto responsibility that the child

may not feel ready for, but then transfer it little-by-little once you see that they are.

In summary, as you practice engaging your child in co-regulation, the main thing to keep in mind when they seem disinterested or not able to engage, is the *role* you have assigned. This is always the place to start. If it is too hard, scale it back and try again. If it is too easy, add challenge by adding complexity or giving them more decision-making responsibility. If you are sure that the role is competent, and that is not the obstacle, then try out a scaffolding method above to encourage them to join without worry.

PART 5:

PEER INTERACTION AND FRIENDSHIPS

CHAPTER 10:
Creating Positive, Successful Peer Interactions

So now this is where all that you have been learning so far becomes real! You will learn how to apply the ideas of co-regulation paired with declarative language to support peer interaction. Or in other words, use declarative language and co-regulation to help your child connect to and form relationships with other kids, and over time, develop friendships. This is everything, right? It may seem hard at times, but you have it in your power to help kids experience success.

I know kids with social learning differences often experience challenges with peers. They may not know the best way to connect, how to get in or join an ongoing activity, how to stay in once they have joined, and how to manage the ups and downs that peer interactions inevitably bring. Communication and interactions with adults are easier. Adults are, for the most part, more predictable. We naturally support kids when there is a misunderstanding or breakdown. We often scaffold or add in the pieces that are missing. But, within kid-to-kid interactions, this is where the rubber meets the road. Kids don't scaffold for kids in the same way or may not be as understanding and patient. Yet we want kids to be able to play together, have fun, be themselves, learn, and grow their relationships. So, how do we get started?

Kids with social learning differences may not know the best way to connect, how to get in or join an ongoing activity, how to stay in once they have joined, and how to manage the ups and downs that peer interactions inevitably bring.

To follow are several considerations to keep in mind as you foster peer interaction across various environments. I'll list them here and then expand upon each below:

Competent Roles
Different Co-Regulatory Frameworks
Authentic Activities
Simple but Powerful Ideas
Recess Ideas
Breakdowns and Repairs
Process Moments
Bottom Line

Competent Roles

Here is the good news. You have the tools already, and now we will talk about how to transfer them to peer interactions. First, (you probably know I'm going to say this by now!) you must begin with the idea of competent roles. You want to set your child up for success with their peers by thoughtfully creating peer interactions in which you child will have a competent role. With a competent role, their attention and engagement will be stronger. They will be independent and more confident, and they will be successful.

You want to set your child up for success with their peers by thoughtfully creating peer interactions in which your child will have a competent role. Starting out, this often means that you are not playing a game by its exact rules.

Once you have a competent role in mind, think about another role that will create contingency between peers in the context of what they are doing. Starting out, this often means that you are not playing a game by its exact rules. We can't because games have a lot of complexity, and if we start with a lot of pieces, a lot of rules, even the potential for loss (e.g. losing the game, not getting one's way, not getting to go first), then we will likely be prompting the child every step of the way, and it won't feel good to anyone. We are going to get into the hard topic of competitive games in the next chapter, but for now, think about how to carve out two contingent roles within a game or activity, and think about what role will be competent for your child (or both children for that matter).

Here are some examples for younger kids.

In my experience, kids love the game Cariboo by Cranium. Unfortunately, they don't make this game anymore, but if you have it, you know how much kids love it (and if you really want it, you can find it used). When playing by the rules, kids take turns picking a card, passing a key back and forth, and trying to unlock a door that matches their card, to hopefully discover a ball. There are several materials in play, and though seemingly simple, there are still a handful of steps to move through.

Now, if you have your child play by the rules, you may find

yourself prompting each step of the way (e.g. *pick a card, open a door, take out the ball*). But, if you let go of the rules, and shape this game a little differently using co-regulation, the kids can be more independent in playing. Kids playing independently with kids is what we want to get to, so that they can form authentic memories of their time together as competent play partners and friends. Through this process, you will also help them gradually learn the rules of the game.

Kids playing independently with kids is what we want to get to, so they can form authentic memories of their time together as competent play partners and friends.

Here is how I do this with Cariboo:

I start by having the kids be on one team, and we don't use the cards (that would be too much). Then, I have the kids take turns passing the key back and forth to open a door (using assembly line and reciprocal co-regulatory patterns). Co-regulation happens as the kids pass the key turn-to-turn, and their roles of "key passer"/"door opener" can be sustained in an ongoing way until we discover all the balls. Once they learn the pattern, I can usually fade back quickly so that the kids are independently playing together—my goal. As they continue to be successful at this level, you can then gradually add complexity when you sense they are ready by adding in the cards.

Here is another example: Candyland. Instead of each child having their own gingerbread man on the board, I use one game piece to start. And depending on what will be competent for the kids, I may create and assign roles of "card chooser" and "piece mover." Then you have contingent roles, they need each other to move the game forward, and you determine how to assign the roles to maintain competence (i.e. who will be most competent as the card chooser and who will be most competent moving the guy around the board). For Candyland

and Cariboo, I also sometimes hold onto the deck of cards myself, so they don't become too distracting, and let kids choose a card one at a time from my hand. Again, as they master the pattern and I notice they can handle more complexity, I shift to place the deck of cards on the board so they can choose one on their own.

For older kids, you can use more mature games and apply similar ideas. Examples: play chess but reduce complexity by using only one type of piece to start as kids learn the moves and take turns (e.g. only pawns, only rooks, etc.), or play a card game such as War, and give kids cards one at a time, if too many cards in their hands would be distracting. Then count to three and have them flip their cards over at the same time (using a parallel framework). Jigsaw puzzles can also be great for older kids. Adjust the complexity to their ability (e.g. 25 pieces? 50 pieces? 100 pieces or more?) and assign roles like this: *How about if you do the top part of the puzzle, and your friend can do the bottom?* (complementary), or *You can find the edge pieces and your friend can put them together* (assembly line). Lego sets can be great opportunities for co-regulation too. You can choose a set that is the right complexity level for the kids and assign roles such as "Lego finder" and "Lego placer," or pass the creation back and forth as kids take turns adding Legos according to the instructions.

Different Co-Regulatory Frameworks

Here are some more ideas. Think about the frameworks for co-regulation discussed in Chapter 6. My Cariboo example above uses an assembly line framework (I hand something to you, you put it in its place). My Candyland example uses more of a complementary framework (we are doing different but related things). A framework I absolutely love for kids to engage in together is parallel. Think of how many things kids (and adults for that matter) do alongside each other in a parallel manner. These opportunities can be bonding. It can also be especially successful for kids because this type of framework often has reduced language demands. Kids can move and simply "be" together, while forming important and positive memories as a team. Examples of things that can be done together might be biking, scootering, running or jogging, walking, swimming, or playing alongside each other in a sandbox or at a water table.

I fondly remember two young friends, Anthony and Michael, and how they benefited from parallel opportunities. I saw them together weekly in a dyad (a peer interaction opportunity consisting of two children only) at my office. Both boys struggled to get their words out, yet they formed a true friendship and bond as their mothers gave them opportunities to develop their friendship beyond their weekly session with me. They took them to "do" different things together. For example, I remember they went on a train ride together at a local park and went to the beach together. Although there was not a ton of back and forth conversation, per se, the boys were connected, happy, and comfortable in their own skin. And they were forming memories of their developing friendship through movement and play.

As evidence of this, I remember Michael's mother once telling me that on a different day they went somewhere that they had previously gone with Anthony. Once there, Michael asked for his friend—clearly remembering their time there together in a positive way.

We never know what will be important, or how a friendship between two children will unfold. It is important we set kids up for success and competent roles, and then practice fading back to let the kids decide how to progress their relationship.

We never know what will be important, or how a friendship between two children will unfold. It is important we set kids up for success and competent roles, and then practice fading back to let the kids decide how to progress their relationship. Helping them feel comfortable and confident in their own skin, while alongside other kids, is the first step. And if we are carving out opportunities for kids to be competent, and have contingent roles alongside each other, we are creating space for this to happen. This is different from if we (the adult) decided on the game, played by the exact rules, and prompted kids again and again to play in the way we think they should. This can be disheartening, lead to breakdowns that are too big for kids to repair on their own, and can even lead kids to form negative memories about peer interaction. We would be going down the wrong path. Think competence. Think joy. Think about forming positive memories where kids feel good about themselves, and good about each other.

Think competence. Think joy. Think about forming positive memories where kids feel good about themselves, and good about each other.

Authentic Activities

With peer interactions, it is also great to use authentic activities. Think of all the things you have now engaged your child in, using a co-regulatory framework. You know your child is competent and successful. Now, do the same thing, but swap out your role for a peer's. You can guide the interaction in a positive way by assigning roles to your child and peer, and making sure you assign them roles you know are competent and then contingent. You are the facilitator, who can fade back as you see kids manage the interaction or the process or the routine on their own.

One example is having another child over for a playdate and deciding to bake together. Think of all the partnership roles you can create between the two kids: ingredient adder/bowl holder, stirrers (each having their own spoon and stirring at the same time), cupcake decorators (I add sprinkles, you add sprinkles, etc). Or try gardening outside or inside: we take turns watering the plant, or I am the watering can filler-upper and you are the watering can carrier, or we pass it back and forth as we water plants together. Or think about planting a new flowerbed: I dig a hole, you add the seeds, and then we swap for the next one. There is an infinite amount of ways to create competent, contingent roles with kids around authentic activities, once you start to think in this way. Here is another idea for constructive activities such as blocks and Lego: I add a block, you add a block (reciprocal), or I hand you a block, and you place it on the tower (assembly line), or I find the right Lego pieces and place them in a pile for you to use as we keep the instructions between us (complementary), or we use the Lego instructions and take turns page-to-page doing the steps (reciprocal).

Simple but Powerful Ideas

I observed this first example with my son, Freddie, and my nieces when they were little. They spontaneously created co-regulation while using a miniature hockey set containing a net and three hockey sticks. In the moment, the kids established their own *assembly line* to get a goal, designed and led by my oldest niece, who was probably 6 at the time. One child used the hockey stick to pass it to another, who then passed it to the person near the goal, who shot it in. I know this is not rocket science, but sometimes naming the simplest ideas help us see them and realize they are the exact opportunities our kids need to feel competent and connected to each other! You could recreate this with your child and a friend, and by naming roles in the moment (e.g. *You can be the passer and your friend can be the goal getter.*), you will increase the likelihood of success even more.

Here is another simple yet natural example that I remember from when Freddie and his cousins were young. In this example, they used a *parallel* framework. The three children received plastic flutes for Christmas from my cousin Janice. Immediately they began walking in an impromptu parade while playing their flutes. I observed Freddie follow his cousins, visually referencing them to know where to go, and they all kept it up for a few laps around the kitchen and living room. Who hasn't seen this type of thing? Again, it seems simple, but the positive peer connection in that moment was great. And, the low language demands of this type of activity demonstrate how authentic peer connection does not require talking.

Recess Ideas

Over the years, I have also had the opportunity to think of peer interaction opportunities for while kids are at school, specifically recess. Here are some examples.

Use chalk. Many competent roles can be created with sidewalk chalk, such as drawing together, playing guess the word, or making a group collage as I described Anna and David doing in Chapter 4. At recess, kids could draw in a parallel, which allows for the forming of memories alongside each other, visual referencing as kids check out each other's work, and idea sharing. Or, you could have the kids use one piece of chalk and create a reciprocal exchange, as they take turns adding items to a drawing (e.g. *Let's draw a face. You two can take turns adding an item.*), or create a complementary pattern with guess the word (*I'll be the writer and you can be the guesser.*). Swinging together can be a positive parallel opportunity that also invites kids to form memories together, as Michael and Anthony did. Or when using the slide, kids could alternate taking turns going down the slide and saying, "Ready, set, go!" (I've often created complementary roles of "slider" and "ready-set-go-guy" that kids have loved!). These seem simple, but when you work to create a pattern around the routine that our kids can recognize and be successful and competent in, you are essentially laying the foundation for kids to be independent. Once the pattern and competent roles are established, you will have a landscape in which you can fade back to allow kids to maintain it on their own. They also will subsequently form positive memories with each other around these shared experiences, and feel good together.

Breakdowns and Repairs

Another important area to keep in mind with peer interactions, is allowing kids opportunities to work through their own breakdowns. When kids are competent and engaged in a balanced, co-regulatory pattern, they learn, sometimes with your guidance at first, to not overstep and take over their peer's roles. As a result, when a breakdown happens, you can fade back and wait quietly for the kids to notice on their own, and then work to make the repair.

Example: a child does not realize it is their turn. Stay quiet, and let their peers cue them rather than you. Or if there is a misunderstanding, let the kids discover this, and communicate with each other when they need more information. This is one of the most important things you can practice with kids. And it becomes much easier for you to fade back once you have established a co-regulatory pattern among peers.

If there is a misunderstanding, let the kids discover this, and communicate with each other when they need more information. This is one of the most important things you can practice with kids.

Process Moments

Lastly, I also want to emphasize the richness of slowing down and focusing on process moments such as set up and clean up. It is okay if you do not finish a game or activity in one sitting, because if you don't finish, you can help kids make a plan to continue it next time. For example, take a photo of the game board for all to remember, and engage the kids in the setting up of the game the next time around, starting from where you left off.

It is okay if you do not finish a game or activity in one sitting, because if you don't finish, you can help kids make a plan to continue it next time.

In fact, projects that span over the course of time are great for kids to do together because it helps emphasize their relationship over time, helps them form memories with each other, and allows them to plan for the future together. A bonus is that these skills are also part of executive functioning, so you are actively developing them too (i.e. planning ahead: I wonder what we should do next time we see each other?).

In addition, setting up a game and cleaning up afterwards are great process moments to include kids. This helps them appreciate the big picture of all that we do, but also there are many co-regulatory patterns to be discovered in the set-up or clean-up of an activity. Example: I'll hand you the pieces, and you can put them on the board, or I'll put the pieces in the box for clean-up, and you can put the box back on the shelf. All these seemingly minor moments are rich opportunities for peer interaction and competent roles. They give kids an appreciation for how things come together, provide new and varied ways to connect with others, and show them actual frameworks that can be transferred to other similar but different contexts.

All these seemingly minor moments are rich opportunities for peer interaction and competent roles.

Bottom Line

Here is the bottom line when using co-regulation to create positive and successful peer interactions: think about competence, take your time, carve out roles, help kids find their balance, and respect and allow their relationships to unfold naturally.

CHAPTER 11:

Approaching Competitive Games

I don't think a section on peer interaction would be complete without acknowledging how hard competitive games and situations can be for kids with social learning differences. For example, it can be upsetting to not get the color game piece you want, it can be disappointing to not go first, and it can be painful to lose. I am sure we have all spent time thinking about how to help kids grow into being a good sport, win or lose, because this is such an important skill to have in life.

In the next few pages, I will share some ideas that I have developed around winning and losing. But as you explore these on your own, do keep in mind what we have been talking about all along - to set your child up for success, even in these contexts, by creating competent roles.

As you place kids in situations that they can handle, they will build resilience. But if we place them in situations where the loss is bigger than their current skillset, it can crush them and prevent them from trying again. We do not need to do this.

For winning/losing games, keeping your child competent means that you do not put them in a situation where they will lose, if they are not yet able to handle or recover from the loss. It is not that you won't ever put them in those situations, rather, you will be thinking about what type of loss or what size of loss is manageable for them right now. As you place them in situations that they can handle, they will build resilience. But if we place kids in situations where the loss is bigger than their current skillset, it can crush them and prevent them from trying again. We do not need to do this.

One of the hardest things for all kids to learn is how to manage the ups and downs of games that have a competitive focus. In other words, all individuals must learn how to win respectfully and lose gracefully. All kids work on these skills as they grow, but for kids with social learning differences, it can be especially difficult.

If your child is one who struggles in this area, try to approach this type of play opportunity and teaching with empathy and understanding.

If your child is one who struggles in this area, try to approach this type of play opportunity and teaching with empathy and understanding. If you stop to think about why this learning is so hard for kids with social learning challenges, it makes sense. Kids with social learning differences have *so* many losses and misunderstandings in their lives. These happen day-to-day, week-to-week...much more than for the average child. Nobody gets their way all the time, but an important difference for a person with social learning differences is that they are not as prepared or equipped to handle the disappointment. Their difficulty perceiving unspoken social norms, making predictions, and appreciating the big picture, along with a lowered resilience due to many disappointments over time, make any loss especially painful for them. In addition, due to known challenges accessing episodic memory (or the ability to remember your own personal experiences that may be relevant in the present moment—a topic I dedicate a chapter to in *Declarative Language Handbook*), it may also be harder for individuals with social learning differences to easily recall their last win, so they truly do feel like they "NEVER" win.

You can help kids with social learning differences the most by understanding the difficulties they face, and approaching them with care, while they work towards building their resilience, improving their ability to predict loss, and overall strengthening their ability to manage loss with grace. In other words, be kind while kids are working to improve their ability to understand that losing a game is expected and manageable, and to stay emotionally regulated. And, as you actively use your tools of declarative language and co-regulation, this will help you.

The goal is to carefully build kids up and help them experience a series of successes in their own emotional regulation, which will then grow over time.

As you enter competitive activities with this compassionate mindset, there are additional ways to thoughtfully approach and practice winning and losing. The goal is to carefully build kids up and help them experience a series of successes in their own emotional regulation, which will then grow over time. In contrast, placing them in less thoughtful contexts where they lose big, can break them. This is not what you want, as it is not good for anyone.

Here are five tips, or thoughtful ways, to approach competitive games that provide kids important opportunities to build their ability to manage loss.

Co-Regulation Handbook

Tip #1: Create many small opportunities which allow for balanced wins and losses

Play games that have many small opportunities to win or lose, versus games that have only one big win at the end. Examples include the card game War, Rat-a-Tat Cat (a card game by Gamewright in which you play a game with several rounds), or even tic-tac-toe (all you need is a piece of paper and a pencil!). These are more likely to be positive competitive experiences because the small losses are manageable. For example, in a game such as War, it will be easy to illustrate this type of idea to your child: *Yes, you may have just lost that one round, but look... you still have a whole deck of cards left and chances are, you will win a round again very soon!* Each quick round also provides the adult opportunities to model self-talk for the kids to then use themselves (*It's okay my card was a lower number. I'll have another turn to try again in a second!*), as well as language of good sportsmanship (*Good game! You won that round fair and square.*).

Kids can manage loss better in these types of contexts because they can see very concretely (in the deck of cards in their hand for example) all the future opportunities in which they might win. They can also see their accumulation of previous wins close by in their win pile, which keeps feelings of loss from getting too big.

Importantly, these types of games also offer many opportunities for co-regulation with one's play partner. As you play this type of game round-to-round, you are likely in sync, can read your child's cues well as you go, and can pace actions accordingly. All these things support their success in handling loss, as well.

Tip #2: Play winning/losing games as a team

Have kids play games in partnership with others so that the loss is not individual. When playing as partners, kids can share the loss with someone, which creates camaraderie and helps it hurt less. In addition, a positive relationship can often support their ability to handle the loss, especially if one person in the partnership is skilled at losing well. Kids could partner with each other, or if at home, different caregivers could partner with different kids. Examples of this strategy in use might be with a game of "Team Candyland" where we use one Gingerbread person as we move towards Candy Castle instead of several game pieces, or with The Ladybug Game by Zobmondo!! We can play with one ladybug piece that moves across the board and together we gather 10 aphids to give to the ants at the designated time.

When playing as partners, kids can share the loss with someone, which creates camaraderie and helps it hurt less.

Tip #3: Kids vs. Grown-ups!

This one is especially fun and builds upon Tip #2. Creating "Kids vs. Grown-ups" opportunities when playing a competitive game is always a great way to carefully help kids get their toes wet while practicing the skill of "losing." Grown-ups can give the team of kids the successes or wins they may need to stay positively engaged, and then introduce a loss when you know the children are in a good place to handle it. For example, play several rounds of tic-tac-toe, where the kids decide together where to place their mark. Give them space to win several rounds in a row and give them time to celebrate their power and connection as a team. Then, strategically beat them, or insert "grown-up wins" when you know their memories and joy of winning as a team are still strong. These are small losses, but important ones because you are gradually helping them build memories of themselves handling the loss well. End with a "kid win" so they walk away with positive memories of the overall experience, and a desire to come back and play (win or lose!) again.

Tip #4: Use reflection and journaling

Have you ever heard your child say, "I NEVER win!" when you know this is just *not* true? With this tip, you will use concrete means to store and recall personal memories related to the truth of winning and losing over time. Find a spiral notebook or journal of your child's choice and start to log wins in the moment and across time. Record information with the child, such as the date and game that they won, so they can refer to it and reflect with it as needed. With this tool, kids don't have to solely rely on what may be imperfect memory. The truth will become evident and comforting over time. Caregivers can say *and* show them: *Yes, you did lose this time, but let's use your journal to remember all the other times you have won!* Making wins concrete and observable in this manner will help kids perceive their personal history accurately, and as a result, build resilience.

Tip #5: Pace yourself

As with the use of declarative language and co-regulation, pace is important here too. Go slow and introduce losses thoughtfully. You want to create a positive forward momentum where the child builds solid memories of themselves as "someone who can handle loss" and as someone who stays emotionally regulated when they lose. If the loss is too great too quickly and the child falls apart, it will only reinforce the idea they may have of themselves as "someone who *can't* handle loss." This is not what you want. Instead, start small and work up gradually to bigger challenges. For example, think about the game Sorry! by Hasbro, and how many losses and disappointments are inherent in the game. This is not where you want to start, but it certainly could be a game that you can work up to over time as you sense your child is ready.

Go slow and introduce losses thoughtfully. You want to create a positive forward momentum where the child builds solid memories of themselves as "someone who can handle loss" and as someone who stays emotionally regulated when they lose.

Mindfully inserting losses at a pace the child can handle may mean letting them win a few rounds, while highlighting or recording these wins for them, before then introducing a loss. When they do lose, and handle it well, highlight this in the moment. (*Wow! I love how you managed that loss. You are really becoming a good sport.*) When the adult times it right, kids will be more likely to see that losing happens to all of us and gradually feel more comfortable when it happens to them. You want them to begin to think of themselves as someone who is okay when they lose. They don't have to like it, but they can handle it. This is what is most important.

In summary, learning to be a good sport while losing is hard work for all kids, but especially for kids with social learning differences for many reasons. Remember to approach kids with empathy and understanding while you carefully work to build their skills in this area. No kid wants to have a meltdown because they lost a game. Support them to stay emotionally regulated while losing by thoughtfully creating opportunities where they are successful with loss, and build upon these experiences over time.

PART 6

PRACTICE

CHAPTER 12:
Practice Sets to Help You Feel Comfortable

Creating co-regulatory opportunities takes practice! Here are a few practice sets for you to hone your skills and become more comfortable doing so. At first, you may need to plan these opportunities and engagements, but the more you do it, the more automatic this skill becomes!

You can download copies of these practice sets along with example answers and suggestions at www.co-regulation.com.

Practice Set #1: Creating Competent, Authentic Contingent Roles

Part 1: Daily Routines

Imagine your child is having difficulty with these daily routines, or you would like to find a way to increase their participation in chores. What are some ways that you could create competent, authentic contingent roles to help them join and then stick with it?

Co-Regulation Handbook

Keep in mind that there are lots of possible answers! And the best answers for your child depends on what you know will be most successful for them. Remember that you start where you start, and then things will grow and expand from there.

1. Putting on their socks
   Your role: _____
   Your child's role: _____

2. Making a bowl of cereal
   Your role: _____
   Your child's role: _____

3. Packing their backpack
   Your role: _____
   Your child's role: _____

4. Making lunch
   Your role: _____
   Your child's role: _____

5. Brushing their teeth
   Your role: _____
   Your child's role: _____

6. Making their bed
   Your role: _____
   Your child's role: _____

7. Cleaning up their bedroom
   Your role: _____
   Your child's role: _____

8. Taking out the trash/recycling
   Your role: _____
   Your child's role: _____

9. Washing dishes
   Your role: _____
   Your child's role: _____

10. Vacuuming
    Your role: _____
    Your child's role: _____

Part 2: Play

You want to play with your child or teach them a new game or activity. What are some competent, authentic, contingent roles that you could create using the following materials? Remember, when creating competent roles, you don't need to play a game by the rules when starting out. You want to think about what will be successful for your child. This is what will help them join, stay engaged over time, and will help you expand their role and add complexity as they are ready.

1. Ball
   Your role: _____
   Your child's role: _____

2. Deck of cards
   Your role: _____
   Your child's role: _____

3. Markers and paper
   Your role: _____
   Your child's role: _____

4. Playdough
   Your role: _____
   Your child's role: _____

5. Shovel and pail
   Your role: _____
   Your child's role: _____

6. Legos
   Your role: _____
   Your child's role: _____

7. Jigsaw puzzle
   Your role: _____
   Your child's role: _____

8. Strategy game (like checkers, chess, or backgammon)
   Your role: _____
   Your child's role: _____

9. Book or magazine
   Your role: _____
   Your child's role: _____

10. Fishing rod and bait
    Your role: _____

    Your child's role: _____

Practice Set #2: Adjusting Complexity

As you use co-regulation and declarative language, it is important to read your child's cues in the moment. You may notice things are too challenging because you are needing to prompt attention and next steps frequently. Or, you may notice things are too easy because your child has mastered their current role and is starting to feel bored.

In this practice set, you will think about how to scale back or change your child's role to keep them competent when things are too hard, and then think about how to transfer responsibility when their role seems too easy.

1. <u>Folding a towel</u> - Your role is to hold one end of the towel, and your child's role is to hold the other.

   Situation 1: This role is too hard for your child. How could you change roles to keep them competent?

   Situation 2: Your child is starting to feel bored and they are ready for more of a challenge! What aspect of your role could you now transfer to them?

2. <u>Making a salad</u> - Your role is to cut the vegetables and your child's role is to place them in the bowl.

Situation 1: This role is too hard for your child. How could you change roles to keep them competent?

Situation 2: Your child is starting to feel bored and they are ready for more of a challenge! What aspect of your role could you now transfer to them?

3. <u>Doing laundry</u> - Your role is to hand an item to your child, and their role is to put it in the washing machine.

    Situation 1: This role is too hard for your child. How could you change roles to keep them competent?

    Situation 2: Your child is starting to feel bored and they are ready for more of a challenge! What aspect of your role could you now transfer to them?

4. <u>Putting laundry away</u> - Your role is to fold, and your child's role is to place the item in its appropriate drawer.

    Situation 1: This role is too hard for your child. How could you change roles to keep them competent?

    Situation 2: Your child is starting to feel bored and they are ready for more of a challenge! What aspect of your role could you now transfer to them?

5. <u>Changing batteries on a flashlight</u> - Your role is to use the screwdriver to open the panel and your child's role is to place batteries in their appropriate location.

Situation 1: This role is too hard for your child. How could you change roles to keep them competent?

Situation 2: Your child is starting to feel bored and they are ready for more of a challenge! What aspect of your role could you now transfer to them?

6. <u>Playing a card game</u> - Your role is to shuffle, and your child's role is to deal the cards.

   Situation 1: This role is too hard for your child. How could you change roles to keep them competent?

   Situation 2: Your child is starting to feel bored and they are ready for more of a challenge! What aspect of your role could you now transfer to them?

7. <u>Shoveling snow outside your home</u> - You have two shovels, so your roles are to be shovelers together.

   Situation 1: This role is too hard for your child. How could you change roles to keep them competent?

   Situation 2: Your child is starting to feel bored and they are ready for more of a challenge! What aspect of your role could you now transfer to them?

8. <u>Taking the dog for a walk -</u> Your role is to hold the leash, and your child's role is to decide which direction to go.

Situation 1: This role is too hard for your child. How could you change roles to keep them competent?

Situation 2: Your child is starting to feel bored and they are ready for more of a challenge! What aspect of your role could you now transfer to them?

9. <u>Watering plants</u> - Your role is to fill the watering can, and your child's role is to water each plant.

   Situation 1: This role is too hard for your child. How could you change roles to keep them competent?

   Situation 2: Your child is starting to feel bored and they are ready for more of a challenge! What aspect of your role could you now transfer to them?

10. <u>Helping your child with their math homework</u> - Your role is to look at their book and read the problem out loud, and their role is to write it in their notebook.

    Situation 1: This role is too hard for your child. How could you change roles to keep them competent?

    Situation 2: Your child is starting to feel bored and they are ready for more of a challenge! What aspect of your role could you now transfer to them?

Practice Set #3: Peer Interactions

For this practice set, think about the presented peer-based activities and the specific questions that follow each one.

1. Pretend play: Grocery store

   What are possible roles in this play scheme? There are many!

   Which role do you think would be most successful for your child to start? Remember, you goal will be to transfer responsibility as they are ready, but it is best to start where each child will be competent and then expand!

2. Word search

   What are possible contingent roles in this activity? Imagine two kids are playing together.

   Which role do you think would be most successful for your child to start? Remember, you goal will be to transfer responsibility as they are ready, but it is best to start where each child will be competent and then expand!

3. Kickball

   What are possible contingent roles in this game?

   Which role do you think would be most successful for your child to start? Remember, you goal will be to transfer responsibility as they are ready, but it is best to start where each child will be competent and then expand!

If you choose to make this a competitive game, what might be the best way to start for your child?

4. Hot Wheels

   What are possible contingent roles between two kids that you could create using these materials?

   Which role do you think would be most successful for your child to start? Remember, you goal will be to transfer responsibility as they are ready, but it is best to start where each child will be competent and then expand!

   If you begin and notice your child is distracted, what are some things you could do to improve their engagement?

5. Making cookies

   What are possible contingent roles throughout the process, assuming two children that are peers?

   Which roles do you think would be most successful for each child to start? Start where you know each one will be successful.

   What do you think would be the hardest part of doing this activity, and is there anything you could do proactively to minimize that obstacle?

6. Checkers

    What are some roles you can create between two kids in this game?

    Which roles do you think would be most successful for your child starting out?

    What do you think would be the hardest part of doing this activity, and is there anything you could do proactively to minimize that obstacle?

7. Physical moving activity together (*walking, running, biking, scootering, dancing, surfing, hiking, etc.*)

    If you were to give your child opportunity to move in parallel with another child, which one do you think would be most competent for your child?

    What types of declarative comments might you make while your child and their peer are engaged in this activity, to help them store socially meaningful memories about their time together?

    If your child is ready for more complexity, what are some elements you could add to this routine to increase engagement?

8. Outing

    What is a place that your child might like to go with a peer, that you imagine would be competent for them?

While there, what roles can you imagine would be competent for them?

In addition to using declarative language to comment while there, what are some other ways you could help your child capture and later recall memories?

9. Trivia games

   This can be a nice activity for older kids, especially if they create the game on their own. If your child were to create a trivia game with a peer, what are some competent roles for them in this process?

   If playing a trivia game using a topic that is challenging, what are some roles that could create camaraderie between peers to offset negative feelings related to competition?

   If you are playing and realize the questions are too hard, what are some ways you could help the kids tweak the game so that they persist?

10. Arts and crafts

   What is an art project you know your child would enjoy and how could you carve out competent, contingent roles within that project while they complete it with a peer? Tip: sometimes before you engage kids in a collaborative activity, it is nice to let them make their own thing first, and then guide them towards the joint project. This way, they have had time to do just their idea and will often then feel more open and ready to be collaborative.

Chapter 12: Practice Sets to Help You Feel Comfortable

How many materials do you think are just right for your child in order to help them sustain attention to their peer and their shared project?

How many steps do you think are just right for your child?

If you realize the kids are fatiguing (it is too hard or maybe taking too long to complete), what are some things you could do to ensure everyone ends on a high note?

PART 7:

TRACKING PROGRESS AND RESEARCH

CHAPTER 13:
Knowing You are on the Right Track

Now comes the important topic about noticing change and progress. As with declarative language, changes do not happen overnight because learning is a process, for both of you. You are learning how to create competent, authentic, and contingent roles for your child in an ongoing way, and your child is learning to trust that you will not place them in situations in which they are not yet competent.

Because you are getting better at creating competent roles, you may notice that your interactions with your child are lasting for longer periods of time. You both may experience breakdowns in communication or breakdowns in what you are doing together, but you are not afraid of these anymore. You now understand breakdowns are natural occurrences, and you calmly support and guide a repair. This is evidence of progress.

You understand breakdowns from the lens of competence and that sometimes it is up to you to tweak things to help your child come back and engage more confidently.

Partnership feels so much better than endless prompting. You know to just get in there and partner with your child because that is what will move the process forward in a fluid and positive way.

You understand breakdowns from the lens of competence and that sometimes it is up to you to tweak things to help your child come back and engage more confidently. You understand what a balanced interaction feels like. You truly feel how you and your child are partners in the process of what you are doing. You feel it, you live it, and you embrace it. Your child does too. Partnership feels so much better than endless prompting. You know to just get in there and partner with your child because that is what will move the process forward in a fluid and positive way. You know this is better than power struggles, prompting, and the negative energy or frustration you had both felt before.

You may also find yourself becoming more comfortable engaging your child in new opportunities and inviting them to learn new things, which includes various aspects of the task such as set-up, clean-up, planning, and recalling. As a result, you can see your child is taking more initiative and becoming more curious and open to your guidance through new learning opportunities. Perhaps you even hear "no" less often because your child is not fearful as you guide them through new experiences. Again, this is proof that they trust that you will not put them in over their head. They trust you will not place demands on them that they cannot meet. They trust that you will always support them to be competent. And because they feel competent, they are willing to go outside their comfort zone and try new things, with you at their side.

When kids do protest, do you now try to figure out what the "no" is about? Perhaps you engage them in the problem-solving process to determine where the breakdown may be and what you can do to support their learning from that place. When you do, you can see that they lower their guard more and more, open themselves up to learning more and more, and you can visualize a path forward in which your child is learning and growing, at a pace and trajectory that is just right for them.

Your child trusts that you will always support them to be competent. And because they feel competent, they are willing to go outside their comfort zone and try new things, with you at their side.

Another indication of progress is as kids become open to trying new things, you find yourself transferring responsibility. For example, maybe at first they simply helped you carry groceries in from the car, but now you are also engaging them to put the food away once you get to the kitchen. Or, initially you felt as though you were prompting your child through their homework or their piano lesson, but now, because you have broken down the process of time management, and have helped them visualize the big picture and perceive the process as a whole, they are engaging more readily and becoming more independent over time. That's when you know you are on the right track.

It is not a quick fix and it doesn't happen immediately, but because you are more patient and understand the process of their learning better, you understand it is worth it to engage them as your partner and apprentice as you share roles, and gradually give them more opportunities as they communicate readiness.

You may also notice that you feel more comfortable guiding peer or sibling interactions. You understand the idea of co-regulation and competent roles so well that you can create roles in the moment that help your child feel competent with peers, such that they engage and stay engaged.

Do you now approach competitive games with a different mindset? Instead of forcing a loss because you think your child needs to learn how to handle it, do you instead approach competitive games with compassion and place your child in situations you know they can handle, with your support, and see their ability to recover from loss improving? If you are using this new approach, then you will see they are becoming more resilient because their ability to handle breakdowns and make repairs with peers is also becoming stronger.

If you find yourself slowing down during process moments where you are in a co-regulatory pattern to pause and simply smile at your child, that is a big sign that you are really getting the hang of co-regulation.

If you find yourself slowing down during process moments where you are in a co-regulatory pattern to pause and simply smile at your child, that is a big sign that you are really getting the hang of co-regulation. You are feeling the joyful connection together when you are in sync, your child is competent, and you are sharing roles.

You find you are prompting your child less overall because you understand how to create competent roles for them. Because they are competent, they are more independent. You transfer responsibility as they are ready, which maintains their competence, independence, and leads to decreased prompting. You understand so much better how this works now! You understand that your child is your apprentice and it is as much your responsibility to guide their learning at a pace they can handle, as it is their job to learn and branch outwards as they are ready.

Overall, you will know you are making progress when you find you understand your child more. You understand that when there is a breakdown in your communication or what you are doing together, it very often is because they feel worried about the expectation of the task. You may know that they can do something, but they don't yet have that same confidence in themselves. As a result, they shut down or flee or protest. This is also known as the fight/flight/freeze response, which I discuss in Chapter 2 of Declarative Language Handbook.

You understand that your child is your apprentice and it is as much your responsibility to guide their learning at a pace they can handle, as it is their job to learn and branch outwards as they are ready.

You now understand this worry from a guiding mindset, and rather than ask them to do more, you tweak and scaffold to find that place where they will be competent and feel comfortable entering the exchange with you, and from there you guide them forward on your shared path. You know that as you engage them from a place in which they feel competent, they will be less worried and therefore able to stay with you longer.

As a result, you show them how learning can be challenging at times, yes, but they are someone who can do it. They can persist, they can work through challenges, and more importantly, you have their back. You are there to support them as they work through their current challenges, while also being their biggest cheerleader as they take on new challenges and roles. They become leaders on their own learning path. You do not prompt, you instead observe them respond to your invitations for greater responsibility.

An unexpected sign of progress is that you avoid activities less because your child is more willing to engage. They trust that you will keep them competent, and support them when they need it, because you are reading their cues.

You realize you have also become good at waiting! You wait quietly as your child thinks and figures out what they need to do within their role. You don't prompt prematurely, but after waiting quietly, when you notice your child needs a little more help, you guide with declarative language or by using other scaffolds. If you've practiced it enough, you'll see this is natural to you now and it feels good.

You realize you have also become good at waiting! You wait quietly as your child thinks and figures out what they need to do within their role.

A less obvious measurement of progress is that when people tell you that you shouldn't help your child with XZY because then they will never do it on their own, now you are comfortable disagreeing with them. You understand that learning is a journey and a process, that the most important thing is to keep kids open to learning, and the way you are now creating partnerships—reading their cues, and honoring and validating their feelings—lays the groundwork for a life of enjoyment of learning.

Finally, one of the most important evidence of progress is that you are also teaching your child how to self-advocate, because at the end of the day, this is what matters. We all are in situations that are hard for us at times. We all need to figure out how we fit in, and put ourselves in competent roles. When we find ourselves in roles where we do not feel competent, we find a way to get help. You are instilling these ideas in your child—specifically, that we all learn from people who have more wisdom, knowledge, and experience than we do. When we feel stuck, it is a good idea to seek out a person who has more experience than we do, and partner with them while we learn and gain more skills. This is what you are teaching!

Chapter 13: Knowing You are on the Right Track

Here is a progress tracking sheet with 13 different things you may notice as you set out to implement co-regulation with your child. Be sure to complete this before you get started to document an accurate picture of your baseline attitudes and perceptions, and then complete it every so often so you can appreciate and celebrate your progress and change.

Date	Not True	Somewhat True	Very True!
I understand the idea of competent roles.			
As I invite my child to join me in a routine, I thoughtfully create and offer them a competent role.			
I understand that when there is a breakdown in our exchange or shared routine, it is likely because my child does not yet have a competent role, or a role that they perceive themselves to be competent in.			
I am becoming skilled at adjusting roles to maintain my child's competence when there is a breakdown.			
I am not afraid of breakdowns and am becoming skilled and patient at making repairs.			
I am engaging my child in more daily routines because I understand how to create competent, contingent roles for them.			
I see my child initiate or accept increased responsibility spontaneously or more readily when given the chance.			

I am comfortable with silence and reading my child's cues in the moment. Our feedback loop is getting stronger.			
I approach competitive games or contexts with understanding and create manageable opportunities for my child to build their resilience in this area.			
I feel comfortable facilitating peer interactions for my child because I understand how to create competent, contingent roles between two children (my child and a peer).			
Interactions with my child feel balanced. I am not taking over their role or over-prompting, and they are not taking over my role.			
We enjoy our time together and I understand that sometimes just "being together" is important and enough. We are forming memories as partners.			
I understand how to use declarative language to name roles, guide learning, and help my child know what may be important in the moment.			

Download a copy of this tracking sheet at www.co-regulation.com.

I am comfortable with silence and reading my child's cues in the moment. Our feedback loop is getting stronger.

CHAPTER 14:
Research Related to Co-Regulation

Unlike declarative language, where there is not yet much research on its use for kids with social learning differences, there is a lot of research on co-regulation. If you search this term online, you will find many resources and research studies! It is well known in many fields, which is terrific. This means I don't need to feel responsible, in the way that I did with declarative language, to make the case that co-regulation is an important concept to think about and use.

Yet, the term co-regulation may still seem elusive to many people, and in my experience, this concept is not used as much as it should be when guiding kids' learning. I would like this to change, but that is my topic for the next chapter.

To summarize co-regulation from a research standpoint, in my own words: many professionals are currently thinking, and for a long time, *have* been thinking, about co-regulation. Many people know it is important, especially in the early learning years.

Some resources that have been especially important in the RDI community include Barbara Rogoff's book, *Apprenticeship in Thinking* (published in 1991) and Alan Fogel's work, *Developing Through Relationships* (published in 1993). These authors and researchers discuss the ideas of kids being apprentices to others, and the importance of co-regulation.

As discussed early on in this book, helping parents understand the idea of co-regulation and create opportunities for kids to engage as partners in co-regulation is a foundation of RDI. RDI has a growing body of research that shows support of its effectiveness. You can find these studies and articles cited on the RDI website (www.rdiconnect.com). Authors include Dr. Steven Gutstein, Dr. Jessica Hobson, and Dr. Nicole Beurkens, to name a few.

I will list more references for you in my bibliography, but I want you know that co-regulation is well known and regarded as important. My goal in writing this book is to amplify this message so more people know about co-regulation, and to break it down in a practical way so that more people feel comfortable using it to create learning opportunities for their kids of all ages.

Co-regulation is well known and regarded as important. My goal in writing this book is to amplify this message so more people know about co-regulation, and to break it down in a practical way so that more people feel comfortable using it to create learning opportunities for their kids of all ages.

PART 8

FINAL WORDS

CHAPTER 15:
Where Do We Go from Here?

As discussed in the last chapter, there is a lot of information available on co-regulation, especially for children age 3 and under. My hope for the future is that more people understand co-regulation and feel comfortable using it to support learners of all ages. It is a positive teaching strategy that seems to get forgotten as kids get older. I have wondered when, or at what age, people stop using co-regulation with kids and start prompting instead. I think caregivers and teachers tend to naturally use co-regulation in the early years (without always knowing that's what it is called), but then at some point we shift to prompting.

My goal in writing this book is for people to realize co-regulation is important, effective, and positive—no matter what the learner's age. As an example, adults continue to learn by partnering with those who know more than they do, who have more experience that they do, and who are willing to share and transfer their wisdom. We do not need to keep over-prompting kids when they are struggling. There is a better way. When we keep prompting kids, all the demand for learning is placed on them. Partnering, as we do in co-regulation, helps us shift our mindset and find balance as *we teach* and *kids learn*. The exchanges become more positive, we keep kids competent, and it helps us, as their guides, be thoughtful in where, when, and how we challenge them. And, when kids feel competent, they remain open to future learning opportunities.

When we keep prompting kids, all the demand for learning is placed on them. Partnering, as we do in co-regulation, helps us shift our mindset and find balance as *we teach* and *kids learn*.

Co-regulation also helps kids internalize the idea that it is okay and important to access help from those who know more than we do. It helps them feel comfortable self-advocating. With co-regulation, we teach kids naturally, in the context of meaningful joint activities, that they do not have to know everything. In fact, they learn it is more important to know how to get help or guidance when you need it. Co-regulation also helps kids learn what it feels like to seek that guidance from someone who is invested in them and cares about their learning.

I also want parents, caregivers, and professionals to understand that co-regulation supports growth in so many other areas of development: self-regulation, conversation and communication, executive function, and the forming of relationships and friendships. It helps two different individuals find balance and common ground, both in the thoughtful work we do day-to-day, and the playful exchanges we share. Co-regulation can be fun! And from a place of joy and pride, we all learn more about each other and the world.

Co-regulation helps two different individuals find balance and common ground, both in the thoughtful work we do day-to-day, and the playful exchanges we share.

Chapter 15: Where Do We Go from Here?

I want people to see how co-regulation helps us imagine and be in tune with our kids' vulnerabilities and challenges. Because co-regulation helps us get in sync with the child, it helps us be thoughtful of the situations we place them in. Through co-regulation, I want others to learn that it is not helpful to place kids in situations that are too big for them to handle on their own. But we can help them join anything as our partners, if we take a step back to consider what a competent role for them might be in that moment or situation. Co-regulation helps us slow down. We become more patient and understanding because we better understand the child's learning style and how they experience the world. Co-regulation helps us stay in tune with kids as they grown and learn.

As you practice co-regulation, I want parents, caregivers and professionals to notice when they have placed a child in a role that is not competent for them, or when they perhaps have not even clearly defined what the child's role is. This awareness on our part is vital. We must realize that when kids are stuck, the change often must come from within us.

When *we* modify what *we* are doing because we realize it is not working, we strengthen the child's engagement, competence, trust, and growing awareness that new situations and challenges are not to be feared.

When *we* modify what *we* are doing because we realize it is not working, we strengthen the child's engagement, competence, trust, and growing awareness that new situations and challenges are not to be feared. They are learning opportunities to embrace and face head on, with the support of someone who understands you. In contrast, when we push too hard or too fast, learning becomes negative. This is the last thing we want. There is a better way.

Using co-regulation to connect with, teach, and guide our kids to independence is a beautiful thing. We can learn to transfer responsibility as kids are ready. And, as you put this idea into practice, you will observe how fluid, positive, and connecting this process can be. As we change our mindset in this way, we can create a positive backdrop from which learning is exciting, safe, and enjoyable for all.

But, as with using declarative language, the change starts with us… one exchange at a time. **You've got this!**

BIBLIOGRAPHY

Aureli, T. & Presaghi, F. (2010). Developmental trajectories for mother-infant coregulation in the second year of life. *Infancy: The Official Journal of the International Society on Infant Studies*, 15(6), 557-585.

Bibok, M., Carpendale, J.I.M., Muller, U. (2009). Parental scaffolding and the development of executive function. *New directions for child and adolescent development*. Spring 2009. P. 17-34.

Biel, L. & Peske, N. (2009). *Raising a sensory smart child: The definitive handbook for helping your child with sensory processing issues, revised and updated edition*. London: Penguin Books.

Binns, A. (2019). Applying a self-regulation and communication framework to autism intervention. *Autism and Developmental Disorders*. 17(2): 34-45.

Braaten, E. & Willoughby, B. (2014). *Bright kids who can't keep up*. New York, NY: The Guilford Press.

Brown, B. (2010). *The gifts of imperfection: Let go of who you think you're supposed to be and embrace who you are.* Center City, MN: Hazelden Publishing.

Brownell, C. & Kopp, C. (2007). *Socioemotional development in the toddler years: Transitions and transformations.* New York: Guilford Press.

Cook, B. & Garnett, M. (2018). *Spectrum women.* London: Jessica Kingsley Publishers.

Dawson, P. & Guare, R. (2009). *Smart but scattered: The revolutionary "executive skills" approach to helping kids reach their potential.* New York: Guildford Press.

DeThorne, L. (2020). Revealing the double empathy problem. *The ASHA Leader.* 25(3): 58-65.

Dweck, C.S. (2007). *Mindset: The new psychology of success.* New York, NY: Ballantine Books.

Fantasia, V., De Jaegher, H. & Fasulo, A. (2014). We can work it out: An enactive look at cooperation. *Frontiers in Psychology.* 5: 874.

Fogel, A. (1993). *Developing through relationships.* Chicago: University of Chicago Press.

Fogel, A., de Koeyer, I., Bellagamba, F. (2002). The dialogical self in the first two years of life: Embarking on a journey of discovery. *Theory & Psychology,* 12(2): 191-205.

Fredrickson, B.L. (2004). The broaden-and-build theory of positive emotions. *Philosophical Transactions of the Royal Society B: Biological Sciences.* 359(1449): 1367–1378.

Garland, E.L., Fredrickson, B., Kring, A.M., Johnson, D.P., Meyer, P.S., & Penn, D.L. (2010). Upward spirals of positive emotions counter downward spirals of negativity: Insights from the broaden-and-build theory and affective neuroscience on the treatment of emotion dysfunctions and deficits in psychopathology. *Clinical Psychology Review,* 30(7), 849-64.

Grandin, T. & Panek, R. (2013). *The Autistic brain: Thinking across the spectrum.* New York, NY: Houghton Mifflin Harcourt Publishing.

Greene, R. (2016). *Lost and found: Helping behaviorally challenging students (and while you're at it, all the others).* San Francisco, CA: Jossey-Bass.

Greene, R. (2008). *Lost at school: Why our kids with behavioral challenges are falling through the cracks and how we can help them.* New York, NY: Scribner.

Groden, J., Kantor, A, Woodard, C & Lipsitt, L. (2011). *How everyone on the Autism Spectrum, young and old, can ....:Become resilient, be more optimistic, enjoy humor, be kind, and increase self-efficacy – A positive psychology approach.* London: Jessica Kingsley Publishers.

Gutstein, S. E. (2009). Empowering families through Relationship Development Intervention®: an important part of the biopsychosocial management of autism spectrum disorders. *Annals of Clinical Psychiatry*, 21(3), 174-82.

Gutstein, S.E. (2004). Relationship Development Intervention®: Developing a treatment program to address the unique social and emotional deficits in Autism Spectrum Disorder. *Autism Spectrum Quarterly,* Winter, 8-12.

Gutstein, S.E. (2004). The effectiveness of Relationship Development Intervention® on remediating core deficits of autism-spectrum children. *Journal of Developmental and Behavioral Pediatrics*, 25(5), 275.

Gutstein, S. E. (2009). *The RDI book: Forging new pathways for Autism, Asperger's and PDD with the Relationship Development Intervention ® Program*. Houston, TX: Connections Center Publishing.

Gutstein, S. E., Burgess, A. F., & Montfort, K. (2007). Evaluation of the Relationship Development Intervention® Program. *Autism: The International Journal of Research and Practice*, 11(5), 397-411.

Gutstein, S. E. (2007). *Relationship Development Intervention® (RDI®) Program and education.* Houston, TX: Connections Center Publishing.

Hammond, S. I., Muller, U., Carpendale, J.I.M., Bibok, M.B., & Lieberman-Finestone, D.P. (2012). The effects of parental scaffolding on preschooler's executive function. *Developmental Psychology*, 48(1), 271-281.

Bibliography

Hobson, J. A., Hobson, P., Gutstein, S., Ballarani, A., Bargiota, K. (2008). Caregiver-child relatedness in autism, what changes with intervention? Poster presented at the meeting of the *International Meeting for Autism Research.*

Hobson, J.A., Larkin, F., Hollaway, L., & Garlington, M. (2019). Diminished responsiveness to parental tutoring in preschoolers with ASD: Implications for the guided participation relationship. Poster presented at the International Society for Autism Research Annual Meeting.

Hobson, J. A., Tarver, L., Beurkens, N., & Hobson, R. P. (2016). The relation between severity of Autism and caregiver-child interaction: A study in the context of Relationship Development Intervention. *Journal of Abnormal Child Psychology.* 44(4), 745-55.

Kedar, I. (2012). *Ido in Autismland: Climbing out of Autism's silent prison.* Sharon Kedar.

Keller, G. (2013). *The ONE thing: The surprisingly simple truth behind extraordinary results.* Austin, TX: Bard Press.

Kim, C. (2014). *Nerdy, shy and socially inappropriate: A user guide to an Asperger life.* London: Jessica Kingsley Publishers.

Kranowitz, C. (2006). *The out-of-sync child: Recognizing and coping with sensory processing disorder.* New York: TarcherPerigee.

Kuypers, L. (2011). *The Zones of Regulation: A curriculum*

designed to foster self-regulation and emotional control. Santa Clara, CA: Think Social Publishing, Inc.

Milton, D. (2012). On the ontological status of autism: The 'double empathy problem'. *Disability & Society.* 27(6): 883-887.

Murphy, L.K. (2019). Approaching competitive games with care: Five tips to help kids become better at losing. *Autism Asperger's Digest.* August – October 2019, 28-30.

Murphy, L.K. (2011). Co-regulation: Creating opportunities within natural environments and routines. *Autism Spectrum Quarterly.* Fall, 12-14.

Murphy, L.K. (2011). Co-regulation: The basis for all social interaction. *Autism Spectrum Quarterly.* Summer, 13-14.

Murphy, L.K. (2020). *Declarative language handbook.* Linda K. Murphy.

Murphy, L.K. (2018). Developing friendships: Tips for creating positive peer interaction. *Autism Asperger's Digest.* February – April, 35-37.

Murphy, L.K. (2010). Episodic memory, experience sharing, and children with ASD. *Autism Spectrum Quarterly,* Fall, 15-16.

Murphy, L.K. (2010). The critical importance of declarative language input for children with ASD. *Autism Spectrum Quarterly,* Winter, 8-10.

Bibliography

Murphy, L.K. (2019). The importance of sharing personal memories to make language meaningful. *Autism Asperger's Digest,* February – April, 33-35.

Murphy, L.K. (2014). The value of keeping things simple. *Autism Spectrum Quarterly.* Winter, 18-20.

Murphy, L.K. (2018). What we say and how we say it matters. *Autism Asperger's Digest,* August – October, 32-33.

Larkin, F., Guerin, S., Hobson, J. A., & Gutstein, S. E. (2015). The relationship development assessment – research version: Preliminary validation of a clinical tool and coding schemes to measure parent-child interaction in autism. *Clinical Child Psychology and Psychiatry*, 20(2), 239-60.

Prizant, B. M. (2010). Respect begins with language: Part I. *Autism Spectrum Quarterly,* Summer, 26-28.

Prizant, B. M. (2010). Respect begins with language: Part II. *Autism Spectrum Quarterly,* Fall, 29-33.

Prizant, B. M. (2011). The use and misuse of evidence-based practice: Implications for persons with ASD. *Autism Spectrum Quarterly,* Fall, 43-49.

Prizant, B. M. (2009). Treatment options and parent choice: Is ABA the only way? Part II. *Autism Spectrum Quarterly*, Spring, 28-32.

Prizant, B.M., (2015). *Uniquely Human.* New York: Simon and Schuster.

Prizant, B. M., and Laurent, A.C. (2011). Behavior is not the issue: An emotional regulation perspective on problem behavior: Part I. *Autism Spectrum Quarterly*, Spring, 28-30.

Prizant, B. M., and Laurent, A.C. (2011) Behavior is not the issue: An emotional regulation perspective on Problem Behavior: Part II. *Autism Spectrum Quarterly,* Summer, 34-37.

Rogoff, B., (1991). *Apprenticeship in thinking*. Oxford: Oxford University Press.

Siegel, D. (2015). *Brainstorm: The power and purpose of the teenage brain*. New York, NY: Tarcher-Perigee.

Siegel, D. (2014). *Parenting from the inside out: How a deeper self-understanding can help you raise children who thrive*. New York, NY: Jeremy P. Tarcher/Penguin.

Siegel, D. (2012). *The developing mind: How relationships and the brain interact to shape who we are*. New York, NY: The Guildford Press.

Siegel, D. & Bryson, T.P. (2012). *The whole-brain child: 12 revolutionary strategies to nurture your child's developing mind*. New York, NY: Bantam.

Winner, M.G. (2000). *Inside out: What makes a person with social cognitive deficits tick?* Santa Clara, CA: Think Social Publishing, Inc.

Bibliography

Winner, M.G., & Murphy L.K. (2016). *Social thinking and me.* Santa Clara, CA: Think Social Publishing, Inc.

Winner, M.G. (2007). *Thinking about you. Thinking about me.* Santa Clara, CA: Think Social Publishing, Inc.

INDEX

Made in the USA
Monee, IL
16 June 2021